T0291830

Calculations
for
Pharmaceutical
Practice

Commissioning Editor: Ellen Green
Project Development Manager: Siân Jarman / Ailsa Laing
Project Manager: Nancy Arnott
Designer: Erik Bigland

Calculations
for
Pharmaceutical Practice

Arthur Winfield BPharm (Hons) PhD MRPharmS
Visiting Professor, Faculty of Pharmacy, Kuwait University

Ivan Edafiogho BSc (Pharm) MSc (Pharm) PhD RPh
Chairman, Department of Pharmacy Practice, Kuwait
University

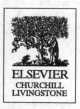

ELSEVIER
CHURCHILL
LIVINGSTONE

EDINBURGH LONDON NEW YORK OXFORD
PHILADELPHIA ST LOUIS SYDNEY TORONTO 2005

ELSEVIER
CHURCHILL
LIVINGSTONE

First published 2005

ISBN 0 443 10019 5

British Library Cataloguing in Publication Data
A catalogue record for this book is available from the British Library

Library of Congress Cataloging in Publication Data
A catalog record for this book is available from the Library of Congress

Notice
Medical knowledge is constantly changing. Standard safety precautions must
be followed, but as new research and clinical experience broaden our
knowledge, changes in treatment and drug therapy may become necessary or
appropriate. Readers are advised to check the most current product information
provided by the manufacturer of each drug to be administered to verify the
recommended dose, the method and duration of administration, and
contraindications. It is the responsibility of the practitioner, relying on
experience and knowledge of the patient, to determine dosages and the best
treatment for each individual patient. Neither the Publisher nor the authors
assume any liability for any injury and/or damage to persons or property arising
from this publication.
The Publisher

your source for books,
journals and multimedia
in the health sciences
www.elsevierhealth.com

The
publisher's
policy is to use
**paper manufactured
from sustainable forests**

Printed and bound in the United Kingdom

Transferred to Digital Print 2011

Preface

Over recent years, the number of UK graduates failing on the calculations part of the Registration Examination has been a cause for concern. There are many possible explanations, including changes in teaching basic mathematics in schools, the universal use of calculators and computers, and the decreasing time available to teach calculations in the undergraduate courses in many UK Schools of Pharmacy as pressure increases for space in the curriculum.

In preparing the third edition of *Pharmaceutical Practice*, edited by A. Winfield and R. Richards, the chapter on calculations was expanded to meet a perceived need. However, space was strictly limited in such a broadly based book. From this emerged the concept of producing a more comprehensive book dealing with the calculations relevant to the practice of pharmacy.

The best way to learn a subject is to teach it—a sentiment with which the authors concur! Failing that option, the next best way of learning is to do. Therefore, in planning this book, we have attempted to include a wide range of self-study questions. We recognize that students start from many different levels of competence. Therefore, we have included some very basic material for those who feel the need. Our experience has shown that it is often a lack of understanding of one of these fundamental processes which leads to problems later on.

In planning this book we have attempted to be comprehensive by including as many of the different types of calculation found in practice as are feasible. However, even in a book of this size, there are space constraints, and it has not been possible to include everything. Indeed, in the chapters dealing with pharmacoeconomics, statistics and pharmacokinetics, only the most basic equations have been dealt with. Students and graduates who need to know more are referred to more specialized books.

Another difficulty in writing a book such as this, which attempts to concentrate on just one aspect of the practice of pharmacy, is that it cannot ignore the broader knowledge of the subject. Some information has been included where essential, but, in general, explanations and the 'science' behind it has been omitted. It is anticipated that readers will have this information from other sources. Where this is not the case, or where there is a perceived need to explore the background to the subject in more detail, other textbooks will provide the information. Mention has already been made of *Pharmaceutical Practice* (2004), 3rd edition, which is the 'parent' book. In addition there are two companion volumes to it: *Pharmaceutics: the science of dosage form design* (2002), 2nd edition, edited by M.E. Aulton, which provides information about the scientific aspects of the formulation of medicines, and *Clinical Pharmacy and Therapeutics* (2003), 3rd edition edited by R. Walker and C. Edwards, which provides further information about the clinical aspects of drug use in patients. All three books give pointers to further reading.

We hope that this book meets a need, and that through it undergraduate and preregistration students will gain the skills and confidence to carry out the calculations required in daily practice. Once acquired, these skills will be a reliable tool to enhance care for patients.

2005

Arthur Winfield
Ivan Edafiogho

Acknowledgements

A book does not appear by chance! Many people are involved directly and indirectly. Pulling it all together has been made more difficult with this book by distance – how would we have done this without e-mail? The experiences, which both the writers have had in different settings, have been valuable in reaching decisions about the material to be included – and excluded.

First, we would like to thank our respective wives, Jean Winfield and Victoria Edafiogho. Jean, as a pharmacist, has made a significant contribution to improving the text and has been able to check for accuracy. Both of us acknowledge that, without the support and encouragement of our wives and families, the time required to produce a book could not have been set aside.

Our colleagues and former colleagues have also had important roles. In particular we would like to mention Dr Kamal Matar, Assistant Professor in Applied Therapeutics, Kuwait University for his input into the pharmacokinetics chapter and Dr Eman Abahussain, Clinical Lecturer, Department of Pharmacy Practice, Kuwait University, for advice on the statistics chapter. Other staff in the Department of Pharmacy Practice, Kuwait University have had significant influence on the authors over a number of years, which has indirectly contributed to the present book, as have former colleagues at the School of Pharmacy in The Robert Gordon University, Aberdeen, Scotland.

Thanks are also expressed to the publishers, in particular Ellen Green and Siân Jarman; their experience, knowledge and ready guidance have made the process much less stressful than it might have been.

Finally, we must thank our past students. As mentioned in the Preface, teaching is the best way to learn. Our students in the UK and in Kuwait have been available to solve many of the calculations. You taught us a lot about the appropriate ways of teaching calculations. We hope that these are reflected in this book.

2005

Arthur Winfield
Ivan Edafiogho

Contents

About this book   xi

1   Introduction   1

2   Quantities and units   11

3   Expressions of concentration   25

4   Drugs in different forms   41

5   Density   53

6   Solubility   59

7   Master formulae   67

8   Changing concentration   95

9   Trituration   119

10   Suppositories and pessaries   127

11   Calculation of doses   139

12   Paediatric doses   161

13   Reconstitution for oral and parenteral use   171

14   Calculations associated with injections   181

15   Other practice related topics   205

16   Basic statistics   223

17   Introductory pharmacokinetics   239

18   Mock registration examination paper   249

19   Answers   257

Appendix 1   Basic arithmetic processes and self-study   297

Appendix 2   Systems of weights and measures   307

References and further reading   313

Index   315

About this book

The aim in this book is to provide a comprehensive and
clearly explained guide to all the calculations which an
undergraduate is likely to meet in Pharmacy Practice and
Clinical Pharmacy. At the same time we have attempted to
include all the forms of calculation which could be
encountered in the RPSGB Registration Examination. In the
belief that it is through practice that competence is gained,
there are a large number of different self-study calculations at
the end of each chapter. Also included is a 'mock' registration
examination calculation paper. It is hoped that this book will
be useful to many undergraduates and pharmacists around
the world.

One of the most difficult decisions which the authors faced
was the question of where to start – what was it safe to
assume was known by readers and what should be covered
in case the arithmetic skills had not been developed (or had
been forgotten)? It was decided to err on the side of caution
and include some basic information. Therefore the early
chapters, and Appendix 1, deal with underlying arithmetic
skills which should be at the disposal of all pharmacists.
Many students will not require to spend long on these
chapters, although there are some aspects which are
essential in pharmacy and should not be overlooked. These
include the use and interconversion of units, the many ways
of expressing concentration and the use of density,
displacement volume and solubility data.

Following this introduction, we have attempted to move in
a logical progression through different types of calculation
which are relevant to the day-to-day work of a pharmacist.
There are, therefore, chapters dealing with master formulae
(which also include calculations for emulsions and

suspensions), the many calculations involving concentration changes, trituration and finally the preparation of suppositories and pessaries.

The chapters then become more clinically oriented as we consider dosage calculations, paediatric doses, the reconstitution of medicines for oral or injection use and the preparation and administration of injections, especially infusions.

We felt that the book should include some other calculations of a type which are increasingly being required. Chapter 15 deals briefly with the calculation of body mass index before developing some of the calculations used in pharmacoeconomics. Full-scale studies are inevitably complex, but an understanding of the principles and methods of calculation will be useful in the interpretation of published information. This chapter concludes with a section on 'business' calculations, including the pricing of 'private' prescriptions. Chapter 16 gives an introduction to simple statistics. Finally, chapter 17 has an introduction to pharmacokinetic calculations. As with the other chapters in this section, there is far more to the subject than can be dealt with in this text. Therefore pharmacists who require more in-depth study, should refer to more specialized texts.

Copious self-study questions are included. It is not intended that every student should do all these questions. If you think you can carry out a type of calculation, try one or two then move on to the next. If you find that you cannot solve them, compare the question with the worked examples in the chapter and try to relate them to each other. Experience shows that once a struggle has been resolved you will feel more confident in future! The RPSGB Registration Examination often looms large in the psyche of students – particularly the calculation questions. It is our hope that, after studying this book, you will have no problems with these questions. The 'mock' paper is in a multiple-choice format like the Registration Examination. Although we have not used this format on the way through because of the space they occupy, you should have no difficulty in arriving at the correct arithmetic answer. Having done that, apply it logically to the options which you are offered.

Information changes and new knowledge becomes available all the time. This book was prepared during the currency of BNF 46. It is recognized that with time there will be changes. This is inevitable. It does, however, offer the opportunity to emphasize that keeping up to date is an essential part of being a professional pharmacist. Whilst you may need to refer to the BNF 46 for the 'mock' paper, in practice you must always use the most recent information.

Introduction

After studying this chapter you will be able to:

- **Understand the importance of carrying out calculations accurately**
- **Appreciate the reasons for the Registration Examination regulations on calculations**
- **Round answers to the appropriate number of significant figures or required number of decimal places**
- **Estimate answer by approximation and compare it with the calculated answer**
- **Adopt a methodical approach to working**

INTRODUCTION

Pharmacy students are frequently apprehensive about carrying out calculations. There may be many reasons for this, including:

- fear of making a simple mistake
- a lack of certainty about the correct way to do the calculation
- a lack of self-confidence in carrying out arithmetic processes
- a perceived lack of ability in mathematics
- 'horror stories' from fellow students.

These feelings may be exacerbated by the Royal Pharmaceutical Society of Great Britain (RPSGB) placing a large emphasis on calculations in the Registration Examination. Certainly it can engender concern in a graduate that they could fail the examination on the basis of a poor performance in calculations.

Despite these worries, it will become obvious when working through this book that most calculations are simple arithmetic, not advanced mathematics and, therefore, need present no difficulty.

Pharmacists must be able to calculate accurately and reliably, having the self-confidence that the answer arrived at is correct. Failure to acquire this ability could lead to serious consequences. For example, if an error is made in calculation of a quantity of drug to be used, the patient may receive either too much drug (with possible fatal consequences) or too little drug (leaving them untreated). Likewise, where the number of tablets or volume of liquid medicine has to be calculated (see Ch. 11), the patient may have too little or too much medicine. There may also be other consequences of calculation errors. If an isotonic solution is required and is not produced correctly, tissue damage or pain can result (see Ch. 14). Equally, an error of calculation can lead to problems if a drug, which was thought to be soluble, failed to dissolve.

RPSGB ATTITUDE TO CALCULATIONS

In the Examination Guidance Notes for the Registration Examination, the RPSGB states 'The Examiners view it as essential that a pharmacist can perform calculations accurately without the use of a calculator. Not only might one not be available, but also any number of errors can be made when inputting digits into a calculator. A pharmacist must be able to look at a figure and know it is correct without any shadow of doubt.' These regulations make it clear how much importance the RPSGB places on the ability of pharmacists to carry out calculations. Furthermore, they reflect the concern expressed earlier, that over-reliance on a calculator means that there is a lack of awareness of the 'order' of answer expected.

Where do the problems with calculations arise?

It is recognized that there are two, in some ways interrelated, problems. One is a lack of understanding of the arithmetic processes and the second a lack of awareness of 'number'. The common cause linking these two is probably the widespread use of the calculator. Why? Prior to the late 1970s, pocket calculators were virtually unknown—the first ever electronic calculator was manufactured in 1963 and weighed 33 pounds (15 kg)! Before calculators, the arithmetic had to be done in one's head, or written down if it was more complicated, or by using log tables or a slide rule. Therefore, students from an early age became fully conversant with numbers and how to handle them—it became second nature. Like tying shoelaces, it was done properly without having to stop and think about the processes involved. To be able to do this, people had to develop a sense of number (see later) which gave them an awareness of the approximate answer expected. This was particularly true when using a slide rule, because it gave the numbers, but not the decimal point. Over the past quarter of a century calculators have taken over, and with this, students have lost this awareness of number because it is not required with a calculator. Numbers are simply fed into the calculator and an answer comes out. The 'black box' syndrome then takes over—I don't know (or care) how it does it, but the answer MUST be right. So whether a mistake is made putting the numbers in, or whether a multiplication should have been used rather than a division does not matter—the answer must be right because the calculator says so! This ignores the 'GIGO' principle—garbage in, garbage out! I remember in the early 1970s a demonstration of an early desktop calculator (about 18 inches square and 6 inches high!). A member of staff was worried that the speed of operation would lead to errors. The answer was that, because it was so quick, it would be normal practice to repeat all calculations. When did you last do that?

In order to reverse this process, it is necessary to (re)learn the basics of arithmetic which older generations took for granted. It is not difficult, but it does require practice—lots of it! This chapter deals with some of these processes which are then applied step by step through the book. There is also Appendix 1, which gives some even more basic arithmetic if you feel the need for it. In doing this the intention is not to insult your intelligence—you would not be reading this book if you did not have intelligence. Rather, it is to provide you with a means to develop the arithmetic skills you require to be competent in carrying out calculations—as a student, as a pre-registration pharmacist and as a pharmacist.

This is a self-study book. The authors cannot prevent students from using calculators; indeed for some calculations in later chapters a calculator will be necessary. However, in the earlier chapters, students are encouraged not to use calculators so that they can develop the skills which are needed for the Registration Examination.

SOME BASIC PROCESSES

Significant figures, accuracy and rounding numbers

Students should be familiar with the concept of 'significant figures'—that is the number of figures to be used to reflect the accuracy of the information being processed. For example, a lap time may be measured in hours, minutes, seconds or parts of seconds. Thus in Grand Prix motor racing, we could look at a watch and say the lap time was 83 seconds (using two significant figures). However, if we look at the official result of the lap time it may be 83.251 seconds because electronic timing was used (five significant figures). Both figures are correct and appear different because of the different accuracy of the timing methods.

The accuracy with which a number is expressed is important. Typically a calculator will display up to eight figures in a number. Thus, for example, if a calculator is used, the answer to a calculation might be 27.364925 mg. This means that a balance capable of weighing to the nearest nanogram would be required. Apart from this being impractical, such a small difference in weight of drug would have no effect on the patient. In other words, the figure is quoted to too great an accuracy. In many pharmaceutical calculations we work to two decimal places (using the most suitable units), although this may be varied with the circumstances. For example, we may be going to use a relatively crude balance giving 1 or 2 significant figures, or an electronic balance giving 5 or 6 significant figures. When carrying out calculations, the answer must be given to an appropriate number of significant figures. The latter is usually the smallest number of significant figures used in the input data. Since a greater number of figures may be produced by the calculation (especially if a calculator is used), it may be necessary to adjust the answer.

In order to reduce the number of significant figures or decimal places, follow these steps:

- Identify the number of significant figures or decimal places needed.
- Select the most convenient unit and convert the answer into that unit if necessary (see Ch. 2).
- Count from the left the required number of significant figures, or from the decimal point the required number of decimal places.
- If the next number to the right is equal to or greater than 5, the last required number is increased by one and the remaining numbers to the right are discarded.
- If the next number to the right is less than 5, the last required number remains the same and the remaining numbers to the right are discarded.

Example 1.1
Round 13.2754 to 2 decimal places.

Count to the second number after the decimal point—this is 7.
The next number to the right is ≥5, so the second number is increased by 1 and the remaining numbers are discarded.
Therefore the figure is given as 13.28.

Example 1.2
Round 29.9114989 to 3 decimal places.

The third number after the decimal point is 1.
The next number is 4, which is <5, therefore the third number remains the same and the remainder are discarded.
Therefore the figure is given as 29.911.
Note this happens, despite the remaining numbers all being large, because the number after the third figure is still less than 5.

Example 1.3

Quote 83.5972 to 4 significant figures.

The fourth number from the left is 9.
The next number is 7, therefore the fourth number is increased by 1 and the remaining numbers discarded.
Therefore, the answer is 83.60.
Note that in this case, the increase in the fourth number means the third number also increases. The zero is added to show that there are four significant figures.

Example 1.4

Quote 40254.9 to 3 significant figures.

The third figure from the left is 2.
The next number is 5, therefore the third figure is increased by 1 and the remainder discarded. However, doing this would lose the decimal point, therefore sufficient zeros are added to indicate the position of the decimal place.
The answer is given as 40300.

Rounding errors

In rounding a figure we are changing it—increasing or decreasing. This can introduce errors if rounding takes place before the end of a calculation. Suppose we have to multiply three figures together, each of which is an answer to a calculation. If the numbers are 0.746, 1.385 and 4.235, the answer is 4.3756443 (using a calculator), which would round to 4.376 (because there is a maximum of 4 significant figures in the input data). However, if the numbers had been rounded to 2 decimal places, they would be 0.75, 1.39 and 4.24, and give an answer of 4.42. Therefore, rounding before the calculation has introduced an error—of just over 1% in this example.

Estimating an answer

Another aspect of the RPSGB examination guidance notes quoted earlier is that a pharmacist can look at an answer and know whether or not it is correct. This is often called a 'sense of number'. There are two facets to this ability. One is to be able to approximate an answer, including the order of magnitude, and the second is to recognize what is a reasonable answer.

Approximation

This is the ability which enables you to get an approximate answer to a calculation before you actually carry it out. The following example illustrates the process.

Example 1.5

In a calculation, the equation to be calculated gives the following numbers:

$$\text{Volume} = \frac{201 \times 2.1}{5.1}$$

The top line (without carrying it out accurately) is going to be about 400. Dividing by about 5 means that the final answer will be approximately 80 (below or above). It is actually 82.8, which can be compared with the estimate of about 80 and it can be seen to match. If the answer had come out as 8.28 or 828, there would have been a mismatch and an error would be suspected. An alternative method for carrying out this approximation is to cancel numbers out: 200 divided by 5 is 40, so 2×40 will be an answer that is approximately 80. Appendix 1 has more on how to simplify fractions.

When answering multiple-choice questions, such as in the RPSGB Registration Examination, approximation may be all that is required if only one of the options matches the approximated answer. In such a situation there may be no need to carry out the full calculation. If, however, there is more than one possible answer, the full calculation will be necessary.

Example 1.5 used simple numbers but the same approach can be used for more complex numbers.

Example 1.6

If the calculation above had come out as $198.3 \times 2.47/4.92$, it would have approximated to $200 \times 2.5/5$, and would therefore have been around 100. The actual answer of 99.55 is in the right order.

Reasonable answer

Perhaps one of the greatest worries which students have is that they will get the calculation the wrong way up and so get a wrong (and silly) answer. In the RPSGB Registration Examination, which will have multiple-choice answers, it is more than likely that the distractors will include the answers generated in this way. Therefore, when a calculation is complete, it is necessary to look at the answer and ask—is this sensible?

If, for example, you find that you are making a 100 mL mixture, but require to add 300 mL of one ingredient, something is obviously wrong! In the same way, requiring to add a few milligrams of drug when making a solution of several percent concentration, or finding that an infusion rate should be several litres per hour, clearly indicates that the answer cannot be correct. It is then necessary to go back and check methods to find where the error has arisen. The process of asking whether this is sensible will help you appreciate the processes you are carrying out. It will take practice and experience to be able to do this, but it is invaluable. Remember also that in many cases you can 'work backwards'. Take the answer and see if you can get back to the starting point by a different route. This is not easy under the time pressure of an examination, but will help whilst you are learning the technique.

A METHODICAL APPROACH

It is not possible to prevent silly mistakes. However, there are a number of steps which can be taken to reduce the chances that these will occur. The following is not intended to be comprehensive, but should help reduce the risk of error for most people:

- Understand the process—what are you doing and why?
- Be logical and work one step at a time.
- Neatly write down the steps—all of them, do not jump any.

- Always ensure that the units match (for example g with g, not g with mg).
- Approximate the answer and compare with the calculated answer.
- Ask whether the answer is reasonable and sensible.
- Double-check the answer. Many calculations can be carried out in more than one way, each of which should give the same answer.

SELF-STUDY QUESTIONS

Round the following numbers to 1 decimal place:

1.1	0.64	**1.5**	7.459	**1.9**	17.5753
1.2	0.572	**1.6**	0.0621	**1.10**	29.971
1.3	3.62	**1.7**	0.9947		
1.4	12.78	**1.8**	1.8576		

Round the following numbers to 3 significant figures:

1.11	4.365	**1.15**	105 371	**1.19**	5006.6
1.12	2.724	**1.16**	1372.13	**1.20**	259.43
1.13	0.3194	**1.17**	823.1		
1.14	24.263	**1.18**	7.835		

Round these numbers to 2 decimal places:

1.21	1.582	**1.25**	1.081	**1.29**	1.799
1.22	0.1470	**1.26**	24.6513	**1.30**	0.5349
1.23	0.4484	**1.27**	0.1316		
1.24	0.009814	**1.28**	0.0840		

Express these numbers to 5 significant figures:

1.31	26.981538	**1.35**	0.63546	**1.39**	3.90983
1.32	121.760	**1.36**	1.6493032	**1.40**	1.4090765
1.33	10.8119	**1.37**	12 690.447		
1.34	1210 107	**1.38**	309.73761		

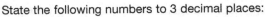

State the following numbers to 3 decimal places:

1.41	74.92160	**1.45**	4.0078	**1.49**	1.00794
1.42	1.37327	**1.46**	58.933200	**1.50**	231.03588
1.43	9.012182	**1.47**	196.96655		
1.44	132.90545	**1.48**	138.9055		

Restate these numbers to 4 significant figures:

1.51	39.948	**1.55**	18.9984032	**1.59**	22.989770
1.52	208.9804	**1.56**	4.002602	**1.60**	0.47867
1.53	79.904	**1.57**	1.74967		
1.54	3.54527	**1.58**	15.9994		

For answers to these questions see page 257

Quantities and units

After studying this chapter you will be able to

- Understand the metric system for weight, volume, length and temperature
- Convert avoirdupois and apothecary (troy) weights and measures into the metric system
- Express quantities of materials in terms of moles and milliequivalents
- Convert between weight and molecular based units
- Convert between metric and imperial measures of length
- Convert between degrees Celsius and Fahrenheit

Most of the time pharmacists will be concerned with using the weight or volume of materials. Technically, a weight is a force (mass × gravity), but in pharmacy weight is taken to be synonymous with mass. In this book, weight is used in place of mass. Volume is the space occupied by a liquid or gas. However, there are other systems for measuring quantity, the most important in pharmacy being the mole, which is based on the atomic or molecular weight of the material. It should also be noted that pharmacists might be involved with temperature and height measurements.

SYSTEMS OF EXPRESSING WEIGHT

The Système International (SI) base unit of mass is the kilogram, normally abbreviated to kg. Often the SI system is taken to be the same as the metric system. However, this is not quite correct because the base unit of mass in the metric system is the gram (g). Students who refer to older textbooks or formularies may also find the avoirdupois system of weight and the apothecary system (also called troy system) of weight being used. The avoirdupois system has a base unit of a pound (abbreviated to lb) which is divided into 16 ounces (oz) and each ounce is made up of 437.5 grains. The apothecary system has a base unit of an ounce (oz) which is divided into 8 scruples or 480 grains (gr). These systems are shown in Appendix 2. Note the grain is the same weight in both the avoirdupois and apothecary systems, but the ounce is different, being 437.5 grains in the avoirdupois system and 480 grains in the apothecary system.

SYSTEMS OF EXPRESSING VOLUME

Equivalent systems for measuring volume exist. In the metric system, the base unit is the litre (abbreviated to L). The litre is also the base unit for the SI system. In the avoirdupois system, the base unit is the pint (pt) which is made up of 20 fluid ounces (fl oz). For the apothecary system there is a fluid ounce made up of 480 minims (or 8 fluid drachms).

ORDER OF MAGNITUDE

In the metric system, the order of magnitude can be indicated by a prefix (Appendix 2). Thus a microgram (μg or mcg) is 10^{-6} of a gram—there are 1000 000 micrograms in 1 gram. Pharmacists must be aware of these prefixes and ensure that, when a calculation is being carried out, all weights and volumes are expressed in the same order of magnitude units. It is, therefore, essential that students can interconvert easily and reliably. Appendix 1 includes a section to help with multiplication and division by 1000 for those who do not yet feel confident. It should also be noted that in the Registration Examination, the RPSGB asks questions dealing with larger quantities as well as the smaller amounts dealt with in dispensing.

Table 2.1 Conversion factors for weights and measures including approximate conversion factors to be used for medicines according to the Weights and Measures (Equivalents for dealing with drugs) Regulations 1970

		Approximate value
1 grain (avoir or apoth)	= 64.8 mg	60 mg
1 kilogram (kg)	= 2.2 pounds (lb) (actual 2.2046 lb)	
1 gram (g)	= 15.4324 grains	
1 gram (g)	= 0.0353 ounce (avoir oz)	
1 pound (lb)	= 0.4536 kg	
1 ounce (avoir)	= 28.3495 g	30 g
1 ounce (troy)	= 31.1035 g	30 g
1 fluid ounce (fl oz)	= 480 minims	
1 fluid ounce (fl oz)	= 28.413 mL	28 mL
1 pint (pt)	= 568.3 mL	
1 mL	= 16.8936 minim	
1 mL	= 0.0352 fluid ounce	
1 minim	= 0.0592 mL	
1 teaspoonful (tsp)	= 5 mL	
1 tablespoonful	= 15 mL	(3 teaspoonfuls)

CONVERSION BETWEEN WEIGHT AND VOLUME MEASURE SYSTEMS

In the UK, the SI system was officially adopted for the prescribing and dispensing of medicines in 1969. It is now relatively unusual to come across the use of avoirdupois and apothecary (troy) weights and measures in the UK, but they are still used in some parts of the world. The pharmacist must be able to make an appropriate conversion if this is required. The principle conversion factors are given in Table 2.1. It will be noted that, for practical purposes, the actual conversion factors have been rounded off. More information about this process can be found in the *Pharmaceutical Handbook* (19th edition, Pharmaceutical Press, 1980).

Example 2.1

A prescription is received for a dose of 30 grains of a drug. How many grams is the dose?

1 grain = 64.8 mg, therefore 30 grains = 30×64.8 mg = 1944 mg = 1.944 g.

Example 2.2

5 fluid ounces of a liquid is requested. How many mL should be provided?

1 fluid ounce = 28.413 mL, therefore $5 \times 28.413 = 142$ mL.

Example 2.3

A patient reports that she weighs 12 stones 6 pounds. The quantity of drug to be administered is determined by her weight in kilograms. What is her weight in kilograms?

Convert weight into pounds. There are 14 pounds per stone, therefore the weight = $(14 \times 12) + 6 = 174$ pounds.
1 pound is 0.4536 kg, therefore
174 pounds = $174 \times 0.4536 = 78.93$ kg. This is approximately 79 kg.

MOLECULAR UNITS

There is another way of defining the quantity of a substance—in terms of its atomic weight or molecular weight (also known as relative molecular mass). The base unit is the mole. For a given atom, molecule or ion, 1 mole is the atomic, molecular or ionic weight expressed in grams.

Example 2.4

Calcium carbonate has the formula $CaCO_3$. The molecular weight can be calculated from the information in Appendix 3.

Atomic weights are: calcium 40.08, carbon 12.01, oxygen 16.00. Therefore the molecular weight is $40.08 + 12.01 + (3 \times 16.00) = 100.09$.
It is normal in official compendia to quote the molecular weight to 1 decimal place when it is greater than 100. In this case, therefore, the molecular weight is 100.1.
1 mole of calcium carbonate weighs 100.1 g.
Calcium, as an element (or ion), has an atomic (or ionic) weight of 40.08.
1 mole of calcium weighs 40.08 g.

The carbonate ion (CO_3^{2-}) has an ionic weight of 60.01.
1 mole of carbonate weighs 60.01 g.

Example 2.5

Copper sulphate pentahydrate is $CuSO_4.5H_2O$. The molecular weight is calculated from atomic weights

$$63.55 + 32.07 + (4 \times 16.00) + (5 \times \{[2 \times 1.008] + 16.00\}) = 249.7.$$

1 mole of copper sulphate pentahydrate weighs 249.7 g.
This will contain 1 mole of copper, weighing 63.55 g and 5 moles of water weighing 5×18.016 g = 90.08 g.

As with the metric system for weight and volume, prefixes can also be used to indicate multiples or subdivisions of moles. In pharmacy we are normally concerned with millimoles (1000th of a mole), micromoles (1000th of a millimole) and, occasionally, nanomoles (1000th of a micromole). Many drug molecules have a large molecular weight whilst relatively small weights are used as doses for a patient. Thus, if a dose were given in molar units, it would result in a very small number.

Example 2.6

Express a 10 mg dose of nifedipine in molar units.

Nifedipine has the molecular formula $C_{17}H_{18}N_2O_6$. The molecular weight is calculated from atomic weights
$(17 \times 12.01) + (18 \times 1.008) + (2 \times 14.01) + (6 \times 16.00) = 346.3$.
1 mole weighs 346.3 g.

$$\text{The number of moles in 1 g} = \frac{1}{346.3} \text{ mole.}$$

The units of weight must be the same for the dose and the molecular weight. Therefore, the dose of 10 mg is converted to grams = 0.01 g.

$$\text{The number of moles in 0.01 g} = \frac{1 \times 0.01}{346.3} = 2.888 \times 10^{-5} \text{ (0.00002888) mole.}$$

This is converted into millimoles (mmol) by multiplying by
1000 = 0.02888 mmol.
It can be converted into micromoles by multiplying by
1 000 000 = 28.88 micromoles.
A general equation can be used to carry out these types of calculation as given overleaf:

$$\text{mol in 1 g} = \frac{1}{\text{molecular weight}}.$$

This is modified for millimoles:

$$\text{mmol in 1 g} = \frac{1000}{\text{molecular weight}}.$$

Moles can be used with ions, but in so doing it does not give any indication of the charge on the ion. The gram equivalent is used to account for this. It is defined as the atomic weight of the ion in grams divided by the valency of the ion. Equivalents are most often used with infusion fluids when correcting or maintaining the ionic balance of the blood. Here the quantities required are less than those obtained using equivalents. As with the other systems, the milliequivalent (one thousandth of a gram equivalent) is most often used. The common abbreviation for this is mEq. The ion could also be a large organic molecule as in Example 2.8.

Example 2.7

What is the gram equivalent of calcium and chloride ions in calcium chloride ($CaCl_2$)?

The atomic weight of calcium is 40.08 and of chlorine is 35.45. Thus 1 mole of calcium ion weighs 40.08 g and 1 mole of chloride ion weighs 35.45 g, whilst 1 mole of calcium chloride weighs 111.0 g. The gram equivalent of the two ions is obtained by dividing these figures by the valency:

Gram equivalent of calcium ion is $\dfrac{40.08}{2} = 20.04$ g.

Gram equivalent of chloride ion is $\dfrac{35.45}{1} = 35.45$ g.

Calcium chloride contains 20.04 gram equivalents of calcium ion and 35.45 gram equivalents of chloride ion.

Example 2.8

How many millimoles of codeine base are there in 1 g of codeine sulphate trihydrate?

Codeine sulphate trihydrate is $(C_{18}H_{21}NO_3)_2 . H_2SO_4 . 3H_2O$.
The molecular weight is $\{2 \times [(18 \times 12.01) + (21 \times 1.008) + 14.01 + (3 \times 16.00)]\} + \{(2 \times 1.008) + 32.07 + (4 \times 16.00)\} + \{3 \times [(2 \times 1.008) + 16.00]\} = 750.9$.

Thus 1 mole of codeine sulphate trihydrate will weigh 750.9 g. Likewise, 1 mmol of codeine sulphate trihydrate will weigh 750.9 mg. However, there are 2 molecules of codeine base in 1 molecule of codeine sulphate.

1 mmol of codeine base is contained in $\frac{750.9 \text{ mg}}{2}$ = 375.5 mg codeine sulphate.

Therefore, 375.5 mg codeine sulphate trihydrate contains 1 mmol of codeine base.

The following are generalized equations when calculating moles and millimoles for atoms, ions or parts of molecules (moieties):

$$\text{Weight containing 1 mol} = \frac{\text{molecular weight (in g)}}{\text{number of moieties in the molecule}}$$

$$\text{Weight containing 1 mol} = \frac{\text{ionic weight (in g)}}{\text{number of ions in the molecule}}$$

$$\text{Weight containing 1 mol} = \frac{\text{atomic weight (in g)}}{\text{number of atoms in the molecule}}$$

$$\text{Weight containing 1 mmol} = \frac{\text{molecular weight (in mg)}}{\text{number of moieties in the molecule}}$$

$$\text{Weight containing 1 mmol} = \frac{\text{ionic weight (in mg)}}{\text{number of ions in the molecule}}$$

$$\text{Weight containing 1 mmol} = \frac{\text{atomic weight (in mg)}}{\text{number of atoms in the molecule}}$$

Conversion between moles and equivalents is made using the equations:

$$\text{Number of mole} = \frac{\text{gram equivalent (Eq)}}{\text{valency}} \text{ and mmol} = \frac{\text{mEq}}{\text{valency}}.$$

Example 2.9

What are the milliequivalent weights of the ions in calcium chloride?

From Example 2.7, gram equivalent of calcium ion is 20.04 g.

Milliequivalent of calcium ion is $\frac{20.04}{1000}$ = 20.04 mg, approximately 20 mg.

Also from Example 2.7, gram equivalent of chloride ion is 35.45 g.

Milliequivalent of chloride ion is $\frac{35.45}{1000}$ = 35.45 mg, approximately 35.5 mg.

To find the number of milliequivalents contained in 1 g of substance, the following equation can be used:

$$mEq = \frac{valency \times 1000 \times number\ of\ ions}{molecular\ weight}$$

Example 2.10

How many milliequivalents of calcium and chloride ions are there in 1 g of calcium chloride?

Molecular weight of calcium chloride ($CaCl_2$) is 111.0.
For calcium, there is 1 ion, valency 2 and for chloride, there are 2 ions, valency 1 in each molecule of calcium chloride. Using the equation:

$$mEq\ of\ Ca^{++} = \frac{2 \times 1000 \times 1}{111.0} = 18.02\ mEq.$$

$$mEq\ of\ 2\ Cl^- = \frac{1 \times 1000 \times 2}{111.0} = 18.02\ mEq.$$

Thus, there are the same number of milliequivalents of each ion. This must be the case because there is electrical neutrality.

As with molar quantities, account must be taken of the presence of water or other solvates. Calcium chloride is normally available as the dihydrate $CaCl_2.2H_2O$ and so, if this form were being used, the calculation should be given as follows:

$$Molecular\ weight\ of\ CaCl_2.2H_2O = 147.0.$$

$$mEq\ of\ Ca^{++} = \frac{2 \times 1000 \times 1}{147.0} = 13.6\ mEq.$$

$$mEq\ of\ Cl^- = \frac{1 \times 1000 \times 2}{147.0} = 13.6\ mEq.$$

Therefore, each gram of calcium chloride dihydrate contains 13.6 mEq of calcium ions and 13.6 mEq of chloride ions.

UNITS

There are some materials, usually from a biological source, where the active ingredient may not be pure in a chemical sense, and so a weight is not a measure of the activity which will be produced. Insulin is a common example of this type of material. In these situations the quantity is measured by reference to an international reference standard. The 'quantity' is then given as 'units' (u) or 'international units' (IU).

VOLUMES

Hydrogen peroxide solution is an aqueous solution of hydrogen peroxide (H_2O_2). It is used as an antiseptic and deodorant due to the oxygen which it releases on decomposition. Whilst the amount of hydrogen peroxide in the solution can be expressed as a weight in the conventional way, it can also be quantified in terms of the amount of oxygen which it can produce. This is called the 'volume'. Hydrogen peroxide solution (6 per cent) is between 5.0 and 7.0% w/v, and is also known as '20 volumes'. Hydrogen peroxide is often purchased in bulk as '100 volumes', that is a nominal 30% w/v (between 25 and 35% w/v) hydrogen peroxide. Thus the volume term is an expression of concentration. Dilution of solutions can be made using either the percentage or the volume measure of concentration.

MEASUREMENT OF LENGTH

Sometimes it is necessary to convert feet and inches into centimetres or metres. The appropriate conversion factors are given in Table 2.2. Conversion is achieved by multiplying by the appropriate factor.

Table 2.2 Equivalents for lengths using the Imperial and Metric systems

Metric	Imperial
1 metre (m)	= 39.3701 inches (in)
1 centimetre (cm)	= 0.3937 inch (in)
1 millimetre (mm)	= 0.0394 inch (in)
1 inch (in)	= 25.4000 millimetres (mm)
1 inch (in)	= 0.0254 metre (m)
1 foot (ft)	= 0.3048 metre (m)

Example 2.11
A patient describes himself as being 5 feet 9 inches tall. How tall is this in metres?

Convert the height into inches = $(5 \times 12) + 9 = 69$ inches.

1 inch = 0.0254 metres, therefore
69 inches = $69 \times 0.0254 = 1.75$ metres.

MEASUREMENT OF TEMPERATURE

In pharmacy practice, there are two common systems for measuring temperature—degrees Celsius (°C) and degrees Fahrenheit (°F). The conversion equations between these are:

$$(°C \times 9/5) + 32 = °F.$$
$$(°F - 32) \times 5/9 = °C.$$

Example 2.12
A patient reports that she has a temperature of 101°F on her home thermometer. What is her temperature in degrees Celsius?

Temperature in degrees Celsius = $(101 - 32) \times 5/9 = 38.3°C$

SELF-STUDY QUESTIONS

2.1 Express the following in metric units:

(a) 20 grains
(b) 30 grains
(c) 160 grains
(d) 400 grains avoirdupois
(e) 2 fluid ounces
(f) 10 fluid ounces
(g) 480 minims
(h) 2 pints
(i) 1 gallon
(j) 1 fluid drachm
(k) 15 grains
(l) 1 drachm
(m) 330 grains avoirdupois
(n) 65 grains
(o) 3 pints
(p) 145 grains
(q) 120 minims
(r) 45 grains
(s) 4 scruples
(t) 370 grains avoirdupois
(u) 7 fluid ounces
(v) 460 grains avoirdupois
(w) 15 minims

2.2 What is the weight of each of the following?

(a) 1 mol of chloral hydrate ($C_2H_3Cl_3O_2$)

(b) 1 mmol of aspirin ($C_9H_8O_4$)

(c) 1 mol of folic acid ($C_{19}H_{19}N_7O_6$)

(d) 1 mmol of griseofulvin ($C_{17}H_{17}ClO_6$)

(e) 1 mmol of dithranol triacetate ($C_{20}H_{16}O_6$)

(f) 1 mmol of glibenclamide ($C_{23}H_{28}ClN_3O_5S$)

(g) 1 mmol of dapsone ($C_{12}H_{12}N_2O_2S$)

(h) 1 mol of amikacin sulphate ($C_{22}H_{43}N_5O_{13}.2H_2SO_4$)

(i) 1 mmol of buprenorphine hydrochloride ($C_{29}H_{41}NO_4.HCl$)

2.3 Calculate the weight of:

(a) 5 mol of apomorphine hydrochloride hemihydrate ($C_{17}H_{17}NO_2.HCl.\frac{1}{2}H_2O$)

(b) 10 mmol of benzocaine ($C_9H_{11}NO_2$)

(c) 5 mol of cimetidine ($C_{10}H_{16}N_6S$)

(d) 20 mmol of caffeine monohydrate ($C_8H_{10}N_4O_2.H_2O$)

(e) 15 mol of chlorambucil ($C_{14}H_{19}Cl_2NO_2$)

(f) 3 mmol of ciclosporin ($C_{62}H_{111}N_{11}O_{12}$)

(g) 35 mmol of digoxin ($C_{41}H_{64}O_{14}$)

(h) 3 mol of ethinylestradiol ($C_{20}H_{24}O_2$)

(i) 50 mmol of furosemide (frusemide) ($C_{12}H_{11}ClN_2O_5S$)

(j) 4 mol of glyceryl trinitrate ($C_3H_5N_3O_9$)

(k) 4 mmol of hydrochlorothiazide ($C_7H_8ClN_3O_4S_2$)

2.4 How many grams of drug are contained in each of the following?

(a) 15 mmol of ergotamine tartrate (($C_{33}H_{35}N_5O_5)_2.C_4H_6O_6$)

(b) 15 mmol of indometacin ($C_{19}H_{16}ClNO_4$)

(c) 10 mmol of methylprednisolone acetate ($C_{24}H_{32}O_6$)

(d) 15 mmol of methylprednisolone hemisuccinate ($C_{26}H_{34}O_8$)

(e) 10 mmol of pilocarpine nitrate ($C_{11}H_{16}N_2O_2.HNO_3$)

(f) 15 mmol of quinidine gluconate ($C_{20}H_{24}N_2O_2.C_6H_{12}O_7$)

(g) 20 mmol of tetracycline hydrochloride ($C_{22}H_{24}N_2O_8.HCl$)

2.5 How many millimoles of drug are contained in the following quantities of drug?

(a) 10 g of quinidine bisulphate ($C_{20}H_{24}N_2O_2.H_2SO_4$)

(b) 10 g of quinidine gluconate ($C_{20}H_{24}N_2O_2.C_6H_{12}O_7$)

(c) 5 g of sulfadimidine sodium ($C_{12}H_{13}N_4NaO_2S$)

(d) 15 g of tetracycline hydrochloride ($C_{22}H_{24}N_2O_8.HCl$)

(e) 5 g of atropine methonitrate ($C_{18}H_{26}N_2O_6$)

(f) 10 g of cefuroxime axetil ($C_{20}H_{22}N_4O_{10}S$)

(g) 5 g of codeine hydrochloride dihydrate
($C_{18}H_{21}NO_3.HCl.2H_2O$)

(h) 5 g of codeine phosphate hemihydrate
($C_{18}H_{21}NO_3.H_3PO_4.\frac{1}{2}H_2O$)

(i) 5 g of codeine sulphate trihydrate
(($C_{18}H_{21}NO_3)_2.H_2SO_4.3H_2O$)

2.6 For each of the drugs calculate the weight of the specified element present:

(a) Nitrogen in 1 mol of ammonium chloride (NH_4Cl)

(b) Barium in 5 mmol of barium sulphate ($BaSO_4$)

(c) Sodium in 1 mmol of cefuroxime sodium
($C_{16}H_{15}N_4NaO_8S$)

(d) Platinum in 10 mmol of cisplatin ($H_6Cl_2N_2Pt$)

(e) Magnesium in 3 mol of flucloxacillin magnesium
octahydrate (($C_{19}H_{16}ClFN_3O_5S)_2Mg.8H_2O$)

(f) Zinc in 4 mol of zinc oxide (ZnO)

(g) Calcium in 2 mmol of fenoprofen calcium dihydrate
(($C_{15}H_{13}O_3)_2Ca.2H_2O$)

(h) Iodine in 6 mmol of levothyroxine sodium ($C_{15}H_{10}I_4NNaO_4$)

(i) Phosphorus in 12 mmol of cyclophosphamide
monohydrate ($C_7H_{15}Cl_2N_2O_2P.H_2O$)

(j) Iron in 4 mol of sodium nitroprusside dihydrate
($Na_2Fe(CN)_5NO.2H_2O$)

2.7 Calculate the weight of the salt required to prepare the specified salt solution:

(a) Sodium bicarbonate ($NaHCO_3$) in 5 mL containing 1 mEq of bicarbonate ion

(b) Sodium chloride ($NaCl$) in 10 mL containing 4 mEq of chloride ion

(c) Ammonium chloride (NH_4Cl) in 20 mL containing 5 mEq of ammonium ion

(d) Sodium bicarbonate ($NaHCO_3$) in 50 mL containing 3 mEq of sodium ion

(e) Calcium phosphate ($Ca_3(PO_4)_2$) in 30 mL containing 1 mEq of calcium ion

(f) Calcium phosphate ($Ca_3(PO_4)_2$) in 20 mL containing 2 mEq of phosphate ion

2.8 Calculate the number of mEq of the specified ion present in the following amounts of salt:

(a) Sodium ion in 25 mg of sodium bicarbonate ($NaHCO_3$)

(b) Bicarbonate ion in 50 mg of sodium bicarbonate ($NaHCO_3$)

(c) Magnesium ion in 25 mg of magnesium chloride ($MgCl_2$)

(d) Chloride ion in 75 mg of magnesium chloride ($MgCl_2$)

(e) Carbonate ion in 75 mg of sodium carbonate decahydrate ($Na_2CO_3.10H_2O$)

(f) Sodium ion in 125 mg of sodium carbonate decahydrate ($Na_2CO_3.10H_2O$)

2.9 Convert the following weights into kilograms to 4 significant figures (sf):

(a) 50 pounds
(b) 30 pounds
(c) 220 pounds
(d) 195 pounds
(e) 130 pounds
(f) 7.8 pounds
(g) 8 stones 8 pounds
(h) 15 stones 3 pounds
(i) 4.5 stones
(j) 9 stones 2 pounds

2.10 Express the following weights in pounds to 2 decimal places (dp):

(a) 95 kg
(b) 80 kg
(c) 21 kg
(d) 1500 g
(e) 42 kg
(f) 500 g
(g) 71 kg

2.11 Express the following lengths in centimetres to 4 sf:

(a) 35 inches
(b) 11 inches
(c) 19 inches
(d) 27 inches
(e) 3 feet 2 inches
(f) 2 feet 3 inches

2.12   Convert the following heights to metres to 4 sf:

(a) 50 inches   **(c)** 5 feet 9 inches
(b) 73 inches   **(d)** 4 feet 7 inches

2.13   Express the following lengths in inches to 4 sf:

(a) 52 cm   **(f)** 93 cm
(b) 82 cm   **(g)** 0.75 m
(c) 30 cm   **(h)** 1.90 m
(d) 150 cm   **(i)** 1.46 m
(e) 2.10 m   **(j)** 205 cm

Answer questions 2.14 and 2.15 to 1 decimal place

2.14   Convert the following temperatures to degrees
Fahrenheit

(a) 4°C   **(f)** 7°C
(b) – 20°C   **(g)** 37°C
(c) 1°C   **(h)** 20°C
(d) 15°C   **(i)** 39.2°C
(e) 30°C   **(j)** 25°C

2.15   Convert the following temperatures to degrees Celsius

(a) 98°F   **(f)** – 10°F
(b) 104°F   **(g)** 52°F
(c) 150°F   **(h)** 78°F
(d) 120°F   **(i)** 40°F
(e) 32°F   **(j)** – 70°F

For answers to these questions see page 257

3

Expressions of concentration

On completion of this chapter you will be able to:

- **Recognize different ways of expressing concentration**
- **Convert between the different expressions of concentration**
- **Use percentages, w/w, w/v and v/v**
- **Express the strength of molar and equivalent solutions**
- **Calculate the dilution of concentrated waters**

Chapter 2 described ways to express the quantity of a single material. Most medicines are made up of more than one material, so it is necessary to express the relative proportions of the ingredients. Many different ways of expressing concentration are used and pharmacists should be familiar with them and how to convert one to another. Sometimes prescriptions are written using a mixture of different expressions of concentration, so the pharmacist must be familiar with these and be able to convert them so that a consistent method of expressing concentration is used. Perhaps the simplest expressions of concentration are as a fraction (for example 1/4), and as a decimal expression (for example 0.25).

RATIOS AND PERCENTAGES

A ratio is the relative magnitude of two like quantities. Thus:

$$1 : 10 = 1 \text{ part in } 10 \text{ parts},$$

which might be 1 g in 10 g or 1 mL in 10 mL.

Therefore, if 1 g of sucrose is in 10 g of solution, the ratio is 1 : 10. Equally, if we have 10 g of sucrose in 100 g of solution the ratio remains 1 : 10.

A percentage is the number of parts per one hundred and is probably the commonest expression of concentration used in pharmacy. Returning to the example of sucrose above we can express 10 g sucrose in 100 g of solution as 10%.

Example 3.1

Express 1 : 2500 as a percentage strength

Let y be the percentage strength. Thus:

$$\frac{1 \text{ part}}{2500 \text{ parts}} = \frac{y \text{ parts}}{100 \text{ parts}}$$

$$y = \frac{1 \times 100}{2500} = 0.04\%.$$

Example 3.2

Express 0.1% as a ratio strength

$$\frac{0.1 \text{ g}}{100 \text{ g}} = \frac{1 \text{ part}}{y \text{ parts}}$$

$$y = \frac{100 \times 1}{0.1} = 1000.$$

Therefore, the ratio strength = 1 : 1000.

Example 3.3

Express 1 p.p.m. as a percentage strength

1 p.p.m. is 1 part per million = 1 : 1000 000.
Let y be the percentage strength. Thus:

$$\frac{1 \text{ part}}{1000\,000} = \frac{y \text{ parts}}{100 \text{ parts}}$$

$$y = \frac{1 \times 100}{1000\,000} = 0.0001\% = 1 \times 10^{-4}\%.$$

It is necessary to make a distinction between different ways of expressing percentages for solids and liquids.

Percentage weight in weight (w/w)

A percentage weight in weight (% w/w) is the number of grams of an active ingredient in 100 grams of a mixture. It should be noted that the ingredients in this mixture could be a solid or liquid, but for the latter, its quantity would be measured by weight not volume.

Example 3.4

How many grams of a drug should be used to prepare 240 g of a 5% w/w solution?

Let y be the weight of the drug needed. Thus:

$$\frac{y}{240} = \frac{5}{100}$$
$$y = \frac{5 \times 240}{100} = 12 \text{ g.}$$

Percentage weight in volume (w/v)

A percentage weight in volume (% w/v) is the number of grams of an active ingredient in 100 mL of liquid. Again the smaller quantity could be solid or liquid, measured by weight, but the final mixture must be a liquid since a volume is being measured.

Example 3.5

If 3 g of iodine is in 150 mL of iodine tincture, calculate the percentage of iodine in the tincture.

Let y be the percentage of iodine in the tincture:

$$\frac{y}{100} = \frac{3}{150}$$
$$y = \frac{3 \times 100}{150} = 2\% \text{ w/v.}$$

Percentage volume in volume (v/v)

A percentage volume in volume (% v/v) indicates the volume of an active ingredient in 100 mL of a liquid. In this case both ingredients must be liquids since both are to be measured by volume.

Example 3.6

If 20 mL of ethanol is mixed with water to make 40 mL of solution, what is the percentage of ethanol in the solution?

Let y be the percentage of ethanol in the solution:

$$\frac{y}{100} = \frac{20}{40}$$

$$y = \frac{20 \times 100}{40} = 50\% \text{ v/v.}$$

Miscellaneous examples

Example 3.7

Express 25 g of dextrose in 500 mL of solution as a percentage, indicating w/w, w/v or v/v

Let y grams be the weight of dextrose in 100 mL:

$$\frac{y}{100} = \frac{25}{500}$$

$$y = \frac{25 \times 100}{500} = 5\% \text{ w/v.}$$

Example 3.8

What is the percentage of magnesium carbonate in the following syrup?

Magnesium carbonate	10 g
Sucrose	820 g
Water, q.s. ad	1000 mL

(Note: q.s. ad means add sufficient to produce . . .)
Percentage (y) is the number of grams of magnesium carbonate in 100 mL of syrup.

$$\frac{y}{100} = \frac{10}{1000}$$

$$y = \frac{10 \times 100}{1000} = 1\% \text{ w/v (i.e. 1 g in 100 mL).}$$

Example 3.9

Calculate the amount of drug in 5 mL of cough syrup if 100 mL contains 200 mg of drug

By proportion:

$$\frac{y \text{ mg}}{5 \text{ mL}} = \frac{200 \text{ mg}}{100 \text{ mL}}$$

$$y = \frac{5 \times 200}{100} = 10 \text{ mg.}$$

Example 3.10

Compute the percentage of the ingredients in the following ointment (to 2 decimal places)

Liquid paraffin	14 g
Soft paraffin	38 g
Hard paraffin	12 g

Total amount of ingredients = 14 g + 38 g + 12 g = 64 g.

To find the amounts of the ingredients in 100 g of ointment, each figure will be multiplied by 100/64.
Liquid paraffin = (100/64) × 14 = 21.88% w/w.
Soft paraffin = (100/64) × 38 = 59.38% w/w.
Hard paraffin = (100/64) × 12 = 18.75% w/w.
It is useful to double-check that these numbers add up to 100% (allowing for the rounding off to 2 decimal places).

Sometimes a percentage is specified but no indication given as to whether it is weight in weight, weight in volume or volume in volume. In most situations it is assumed that solids in liquids are percentage weight in volume and liquids in liquids are percentage volume in volume.

PARTS

When active ingredients are included in equal amounts, or simple ratios, rather than using percentages the prescriber may indicate the quantities in parts.

Example 3.11

℞

Salicylic acid	3 parts
Sublimed sulphur	3 parts
Oily cream	to 100 parts

This means that there will be equal amounts (weights because they are solids) of salicylic acid and sublimed sulphur made up to final weight with oily cream. In order to calculate the quantities required this could be rewritten as:

Salicylic acid	3% w/w
Sublimed sulphur	3% w/w
Oily cream	to 100% w/w

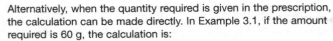

Alternatively, when the quantity required is given in the prescription, the calculation can be made directly. In Example 3.1, if the amount required is 60 g, the calculation is:

Salicylic acid $3 \times 60/100 = 1.8$ g.
Sublimed sulphur $3 \times 60/100 = 1.8$ g.
Oily cream $(100 - 6) \times 60/100 = 56.4$ g.

(Note: check the answer—the quantities should add up to 60 g).

Concentrated waters

Liquid preparations for oral use are often flavoured to make them more palatable for the patient. In extemporaneously prepared products the flavouring is frequently a flavoured water, e.g. peppermint water, anise water. These flavoured waters are available in a concentrated form and are either used as such, or are diluted to provide the vehicle for the preparation. All concentrated waters have the same dilution factor, i.e. 1 part of concentrate plus 39 parts of water to give 40 parts of flavoured water.

Example 3.12
In 200 mL of a particular suspension there is 100 mL of peppermint water. The peppermint water is only available as concentrated peppermint water. The dilution factor 1 part + 39 parts is used:

  1 mL concentrate + 39 mL water = 40 mL peppermint water.

If 40 mL of peppermint water contains 1 mL of concentrated peppermint water, then 100 mL of peppermint water will contain 2.5 mL of concentrated peppermint water. Therefore to 2.5 mL of concentrated peppermint water is added 97.5 mL of water to produce the 100 mL of peppermint water required.

MOLAR AND EQUIVALENT SOLUTIONS

Moles and equivalents are expressions of quantity. Therefore, they can become part of an expression of a concentration in a mixture. In pharmacy this is always in a volume, normally expressed as mmol/mL, mmol/L, μmol/L or mEq/L. A 1 molar solution contains 1 mole of material dissolved in 1 litre. From this starting point it is possible to calculate the amount of material required for different volumes or different strengths of solution. Some examples of these follow.

Example 3.13

Calculate the number of moles (molarity) of a solution if it contains 117 g of sodium chloride (NaCl) in 1 L of solution. (Atomic weights are given in Appendix 3)

Molecular weight of NaCl = 22.99 + 35.45 = 58.44.

Therefore, 58.44 g of NaCl in 1 litre is equivalent to 1 mole (1 mol) in solution.
Number of moles of NaCl = 117/58.44 = 2.0 mol.

Example 3.14

Calculate the number of milligrams of sodium hydroxide (NaOH) to be dissolved in 1 L of water to give a concentration of 10 mmol

Molecular weight of NaOH = 22.99 + 16.00 + 1.008 = 40.00.

Therefore, 1 mole weighs 40.0 g. 1 mmol weighs 40 mg
1 millimole/L solution = 40 mg in 1 L; therefore 10 mmol = 400 mg in 1 L.

Example 3.15

Express 111 mg of calcium chloride ($CaCl_2$) in 1 L of solution as millimoles

Molecular weight of $CaCl_2$ = Ca + (2 × Cl) = 40.08 + (2 × 35.45) = 40.08 + 70.90 = 110.98 g

This is 111.0 to four significant figures (the accuracy to which the atomic weights were quoted).
1 mole of $CaCl_2$ is 111 g, which is to be dissolved in 1 L.
To convert mole to millimoles, multiply by 1000.
Therefore, 111 mg of $CaCl_2$ = 1 mmol in 1 L.

Example 3.16

Normal saline is 0.9% sodium chloride in water. Calculate the number of moles in 1 L of normal saline

Sodium chloride is NaCl, which has a molecular weight of 58.44.
Therefore a 1 molar solution contains 58.44 g dissolved in 1 L.
Normal saline is a 0.9% w/v solution, that is 9 g in 1 L.
Let the number of moles of sodium chloride be x. Therefore:

$$x = \frac{9 \times 1}{58.44} = 0.154 \text{ mol}$$

The answer could also be expressed in units of mmol/L by multiplying by 1000:

$$0.154 \times 1000 = 154 \text{ mmol/L}$$

Normal saline contains 154 mmol/L.

The calculation can be simplified by using an equation for converting a percentage strength to mmol/L:

$$\text{mmol/L} = \frac{\text{percentage strength} \times 10\,000}{\text{mg of substance in 1 mmol}}$$

Thus, substituting:

$$\text{mmol/L of sodium chloride} = \frac{0.9 \times 10\,000}{58.44} = 154.0 \text{ mmol/L}.$$

Example 3.17

How many mmol of sodium chloride are contained in 250 mL of normal saline?

From example 3.16 we know that 1 L of normal saline contains 154 mmol of sodium chloride. Therefore, 250 mL of normal saline will contain:

$$\frac{250 \times 154}{1000} = 38.5 \text{ mmol sodium chloride}.$$

Example 3.18

Calcium chloride injection contains 100 mg/mL. How many mmol of calcium is contained in 1 mL?

The molecular weight of calcium chloride dihydrate ($CaCl_2.2H_2O$) is 147.0. Therefore 1 mole contains 147.0 g $CaCl_2.H_2O$ and 40.08 g calcium. 100 mg calcium chloride contains:

$$\frac{100 \times 40.08}{147.0} = 27.26 \text{ mg of calcium ions}.$$

To find the number of moles of calcium, y, in 1 mL:

$$y = \frac{\text{wt of calcium (in g)} \times \text{volume (in mL)}}{\text{atomic weight of calcium}}$$

$$y = \frac{0.02726 \times 1}{40.08} = 6.8 \times 10^{-4}$$

This can be converted to millimoles,
$6.8 \times 10^{-4} \times 1000 = 0.68$ mmol/mL, or converted to micromole
$6.8 \times 10^{-4} \times 1000\,000 = 680$ μmol/mL.

It is not necessary to do this calculation in two stages, because the weight of calcium need not be calculated. Instead, the two stages can be combined using the equation:

$$\text{Number of mmol} = \frac{1000 \times \text{weight (in g)}}{\text{molecular weight}}$$

Therefore:

$$\text{Number of mmol} = \frac{1000 \times 0.1}{147.0} = 0.68.$$

Example 3.19

A prescription is received for 500 mL of infusion containing 60 mmol potassium chloride. What weight of potassium chloride is required?

Molecular weight of potassium chloride is 74.55.
60 mmol = 0.060 mol.
Weight of potassium chloride required = 0.060 × 74.55 = 4.473 g.

Example 3.20

Calculate the quantities in mmol of each ion in 1 L of Ringer's Solution for Injection.

Ringer's Solution for Injection has the following formula:

Calcium chloride (dihydrate)	322 microgram/mL
Potassium chloride	300 microgram/mL
Sodium chloride	8.6 mg/mL

Convert these to weights in g/L (multiply by 1000 for working in moles), and finding molecular weights:

	Weight in 1 L	Molecular weight
Calcium chloride (dihydrate)	0.322 g	147.0
Potassium chloride	0.300 g	74.55
Sodium chloride	8.6 g	58.44

The weights can be converted into millimoles using the equation:

$$\text{mmol} = \frac{1000 \times \text{number of ions} \times \text{weight (g)}}{\text{molecular weight}}$$

mmol of calcium in calcium chloride (dihydrate)	2.19
mmol of potassium in potassium chloride	4.02
mmol of sodium in sodium chloride	147.16

Potassium, sodium and chloride are monovalent, so there are equal numbers of anions and cations in the salt. However, calcium chloride has two chloride ions for each calcium ion. Therefore there are 2.19 mmol of calcium and 4.38 mmol of chloride ions. Chloride ions are contributed from all three salts, therefore the total chloride content is obtained by addition of the individual contributions:

Chloride ions = 4.38 + 4.02 + 147.16 = 155.56 mmol.

Therefore, rounding the figures to 1 decimal place, the answer to the question is:

Calcium 2.2 mmol, potassium 4.0 mmol, sodium 147.2 mmol and chloride 155.6 mmol.

Example 3.21

A patient has a blood test which shows a fasting glucose value of 5.8 mmol/L. What is this expressed as a percentage?

Glucose (dextrose) normally occurs as a monohydrate, but, because the question is asking how much of the glucose is in solution, the hydrate can be ignored. Therefore, the molecular weight of glucose ($C_6H_{12}O_6$) is 180.2.

The following equation can be used:

$$\text{Percentage (w/v)} = \frac{\text{mg of substance containing 1 mmol} \times \text{mmol/L}}{10\ 000}$$

Substituting:

$$\text{Percentage (w/v)} = \frac{180.2 \times 5.8}{10\ 000} = 0.10\%\ \text{(w/v)}.$$

SELF-STUDY QUESTIONS

3.1 Express the following concentrations as a percentage (to 2 significant figures), stating where appropriate w/w, w/v or v/v:

(a) 1.0 mL in 25 mL
(b) 0.1 mL in 10 mL
(c) 1 g in 220 mL
(d) 1 g in 335 mL
(e) 4 parts per million
(f) 25 parts per million
(g) 110 mg of sodium chloride in 100 mL
(h) 50 mg of potassium chloride in 90 mL
(i) 0.3 mL in 2.5 mL
(j) 90 mg of potassium chloride in 110 mL
(k) 1 g in 520 mL
(l) 750 parts per million
(m) 0.2 mL in 1.3 mL
(n) 1 g in 72 mL
(o) 120 mg of sodium chloride in 220 mL
(p) 0.4 mL in 3.2 mL
(q) 3600 parts per million
(r) 2 g in 630 mL
(s) 55 parts per million

(t) 0.15 mL in 13 mL
(u) 50 mg of sodium chloride in 120 mL
(v) 865 parts per million
(w) 0.6 mL in 58 mL
(x) 100 mg in 940 mL
(y) 65 mg of sodium chloride in 45 mL

3.2 How much sodium bicarbonate is required to prepare each of the following solutions? (To 2 decimal places)

(a) 10 mL of 1 in 10 solution   **(f)** 60 mL of 1 in 45 solution
(b) 20 mL of 1 in 15 solution   **(g)** 15 mL of 1 in 60 solution
(c) 200 mL of 1 in 35 solution   **(h)** 90 mL of 1 in 70 solution
(d) 40 mL of 1 in 55 solution   **(i)** 300 mL of 1 in 90 solution
(e) 30 mL of 1 in 25 solution

3.3 Express as '1 part in . . . parts' the following percentages:

(a) 0.025% w/w   **(e)** 0.0045% w/w
(b) 0.045% w/w   **(f)** 0.07% w/w
(c) 0.055% w/w   **(g)** 0.08% w/w
(d) 0.0025% w/w

3.4 Calculate the percentage of each ingredient in the following ointments:

(a)	Hard paraffin	7	**(d)**	Hard paraffin	10
	Soft paraffin	14		Soft paraffin	40
	Liquid paraffin	8		Liquid paraffin	8
(b)	Hard paraffin	8	**(e)**	Hard paraffin	10
	Soft paraffin	40		Soft paraffin	44
	Liquid paraffin	12		Liquid paraffin	8
(c)	Hard paraffin	8	**(f)**	Hard paraffin	12
	Soft paraffin	44		Soft paraffin	36
	Liquid paraffin	14		Liquid paraffin	14

3.5 Convert the following percentages to mg/mL:

(a) 0.15% w/v   **(c)** 0.4% w/v
(b) 0.25% w/v   **(d)** 0.65% w/v

(e) 0.8% w/v	**(h)** 1.8% w/v
(f) 0.9% w/v	**(i)** 2.2% w/v
(g) 1.2% w/v	**(j)** 2.6% w/v

3.6 What weight of lactose is required to make each solution? (State in g to the nearest 10 mg)

(a) 10 mL of 2% w/v solution

(b) 1 mL of 3% w/v solution

(c) 5 mL of 2.6% w/v solution

(d) 50 mL of 3.2% w/v solution

(e) 15 mL of 4.2% w/v solution

(f) 25 mL of 4.8% w/v solution

(g) 60 mL of 5.2% w/v solution

(h) 70 mL of 3.0% w/v solution

(i) 40 mL of 2.1% w/v solution

(j) 80 mL of 3.0% w/v solution

(k) 90 mL of 1.3% w/v solution

3.7 Convert the following to a percentage (to 2 significant figures), stating whether w/w, w/v or v/v:

(a) 0.8 mg/mL

(b) 1.2 mg/mL

(c) 250 mg/5 mL

(d) 29 mg/5 mL

(e) 2.5 mg/mL

(f) 100 microgram/5 mL

(g) 150 mg of powder is made up to 90 g

(h) 15 mg of powder is made up to 200 g

(i) 15 mg/mL

(j) 200 mg of powder is made up to 120 g

(k) 3.0 mg/mL

(l) 300 mg of powder is made up to 50 g

(m) 640 mg/10 mL

(n) 3.4 mg/10 mL

(o) 450 mg of powder is made up to 25 g

(p) 190 mg/mL

(q) 390 mg/15 mL

(r) 45 mg of powder is made up to 90 g

(s) 200 mg/5 mL
(t) 2.2 mg/mL
(u) 360 mg/5 mL
(v) 1.6 g/5 mL
(w) 3 g of powder is made up to 120 g

3.8 How many milligrams of drug are required to prepare the following mixtures?

(a) 25 g of a 0.8% w/w mixture
(b) 90 g of a 0.33% w/w mixture
(c) 180 g of a 0.17% w/w mixture
(d) 75 g of a 0.6% w/w mixture
(e) 20 g of a 2.25% w/w mixture
(f) 50 g of a 0.3% w/w mixture
(g) 45 g of a 1.7% w/w mixture
(h) 30 g of a 0.5% w/w mixture
(i) 80 g of a 0.25% w/w mixture
(j) 120 g of a 0.17% w/w mixture

3.9 Calculate the percentage w/w of each ingredient in the following ointments:

(a)
Resorcinol	5 parts
Precipitated sulphur	10 parts
Zinc oxide	40 parts
Emulsifying ointment	45 parts

(b)
Calamine	7 parts
Arachis oil	30 parts
Emulsifying wax	6 parts
Water	to 100 parts

(c)
Starch	7 parts
Zinc oxide	8 parts
Olive oil	2 parts
Wool fat	3 parts

(d)
Chlorhexidine gluconate 20% solution	10 parts
Cetomacrogol emulsifying wax	50 parts
Liquid paraffin	20 parts
Water	120 parts

(e) Wool fat .... 5 parts
Hard paraffin .... 2.5 parts
Cetostearyl alcohol .... 7.5 parts
Soft paraffin .... 85 parts

(f) Ichthammol .... 2.5 parts
Cetostearyl alcohol .... 1.5 parts
Wool fat .... 5 parts
Zinc cream .... to 50 parts

3.10. Express as a percentage (to 2 decimal places) each of the following, stating w/w, w/v or v/v where appropriate:

(a) 150 mg of powder is made up to 30 g
(b) 170 mg of potassium chloride in 90 mL
(c) 6600 parts per million
(d) 5 g in 830 mL
(e) 0.4 mL in 28 mL
(f) 2.8 mg/mL
(g) 140 mg/5 mL
(h) 1000 parts per million
(i) 150 mg of sodium chloride in 110 mL
(j) 3.6 mg/mL
(k) 300 mg of powder is made up to 200 g
(l) 1 g in 450 mL
(m) 220 mg/5 mL
(n) 0.3 mL in 31 mL
(o) 800 mg of sodium chloride in 120 mL
(p) 0.6 mL in 90 mL
(q) 450 mg of powder is made up to 30 g

3.11 In preparing an IV infusion, you have a solution containing 2 g/mL of the specified drug. What volume must be added to a 500 mL infusion to provide the indicated total dose? (To 2 decimal places)

(a) 10 mmol adrenaline hydrochloride (epinephrine hydrochloride) ($C_9H_{13}NO_3.HCl$)
(b) 15 mmol adrenaline acid tartrate (epinephrine bitartrate) ($C_9H_{13}NO_3.C_4H_6O_6$)
(c) 30 mmol cefotaxime sodium ($C_{16}H_{16}N_5NaO_7S_2$)

(d) 10 mmol chloramphenicol ($C_{11}H_{12}Cl_2N_2O_5$)
(e) 12 mmol chloramphenicol ($C_{11}H_{12}Cl_2N_2O_5$)
(f) 20 mmol cortisone ($C_{21}H_{28}O_5$)
(g) 10 mmol erythromycin ($C_{37}H_{67}NO_{13}$)
(h) 20 mmol furosemide (frusemide) ($C_{12}H_{11}ClN_2O_5S$)
(i) 25 mmol cefuroxime axetil ($C_{20}H_{22}N_4O_{10}S$)

3.12 What is the concentration, in % w/v, of the following solutions (to 2 decimal places)?

(a) Potassium chloride (KCl) containing 1 mEq in 10 mL
(b) Ammonium chloride (NH_4Cl) containing 1 mEq in 5 mL
(c) Sodium bicarbonate ($NaHCO_3$) containing 2 mEq in 20 mL
(d) Sodium sulphate (Na_2SO_4) containing 1 mEq in 50 mL
(e) Sodium sulphate (Na_2SO_4) containing 5 mEq in 10 mL
(f) Calcium phosphate ($Ca_3(PO_4)_2$) containing 2 mEq in 10 mL

3.13 Calculate the number of mEq in the following injection solutions:

(a) 10 mL of 2.0% w/v sodium chloride (NaCl)
(b) 5 mL of 0.9% w/v sodium chloride (NaCl)
(c) 15 mL of 1.0% w/v sodium bicarbonate ($NaHCO_3$)
(d) 5 mL of 0.9% w/v calcium chloride ($CaCl_2$)
(e) 10 mL of 1.0% w/v magnesium chloride ($MgCl_2$)

For answers to these questions see page 259

Drugs in different forms

After studying this chapter you will be able to:

- Appreciate that the same drug can exist in different chemical forms
- Recognize that the amount of drug can differ in its different chemical forms
- Calculate the amount of drug in different chemical forms
- Handle the calculations associated with the legal classification of some drugs
- Recognize and allow for different levels of hydration in some drugs

Drug molecules can be adapted to form different salts, esters and other complexes. There are many reasons for this, including, for example, controlling the solubility and/or partition coefficient. Each of the different forms has a different molecular weight and so the same weight of drug will not contain the same amount of drug. This can be very significant in ensuring correct dosing of the patient. In addition, a number of drugs form different solvates, the commonest of which are the hydrates. Normally there is one particular hydrate which occurs under normal conditions, but there are a few situations where different levels of hydration can be encountered. The presence or absence of water in the molecule will also affect the amount of drug in a given weight.

A further important aspect of this subject concerns the legal implications of the different forms. A look through the legal classification of drugs will show that there are a significant number where their legal classification is dependent on the concentration of a drug species, as opposed to the concentration of a derivative such as a salt or ester.

In this chapter we will consider each of these groups separately, although the arithmetic involved is essentially the same for each, using simple proportion.

CALCULATIONS INVOLVING SALTS

Example 4.1

Diclofenac tablets contain 50 mg of diclofenac sodium. What is the weight of diclofenac which is equivalent? (Answer to 4 significant figures)

Molecular weight of diclofenac ($C_{14}H_{11}Cl_2NO_2$) = 296.1, diclofenac sodium ($C_{14}H_{10}Cl_2NNaO_2$) = 318.1.

Let y be the weight of diclofenac equivalent to 50 mg diclofenac sodium. Using proportion:

$$\frac{318.1}{296.1} = \frac{50}{y}$$

Therefore:

$$y = \frac{296.1 \times 50}{318.1} = 46.54 \text{ mg.}$$

Example 4.2

Calculate the weights of pilocarpine hydrochloride and pilocarpine nitrate equivalent to 100 mg pilocarpine. (Answer to 4 significant figures)

Molecular weights: pilocarpine ($C_{11}H_{16}N_2O_2$) = 208.3; pilocarpine hydrochloride ($C_{11}H_{16}N_2O_2.HCl$) = 244.7; pilocarpine nitrate ($C_{11}H_{16}N_2O_2.HNO_3$ = 271.3).

Let y be the amount of pilocarpine hydrochloride and z be the amount of pilocarpine nitrate equivalent to 100 mg of pilocarpine base. Using proportion:

Pilocarpine hydrochloride:

$$\frac{208.3}{244.7} = \frac{100}{y} \text{ , therefore } y = \frac{100 \times 244.7}{208.3} = 117.5 \text{ mg}$$

Pilocarpine nitrate:

$$\frac{208.3}{271.3} = \frac{100}{z} \text{ , therefore } z = \frac{100 \times 271.3}{208.3} = 130.2 \text{ mg.}$$

Example 4.3

What is the iron content of a 322 mg tablet of ferrous fumarate (Fersaday®)?

Molecular weight of ferrous fumarate $C_4H_2FeO_4$ = 169.9, atomic weight of iron = 55.85.

Let y be the weight of iron in 322 mg of ferrous fumarate. Using proportion:

$$\frac{169.9}{55.85} = \frac{322}{y} \text{ , therefore } y = \frac{322 \times 55.85}{169.9} = 105.8 \text{ mg iron.}$$

Note: the BNF gives the equivalence as 100 mg iron.

CALCULATIONS INVOLVING ESTERS AND OTHER COMPLEXES

Example 4.4

Tablets contain 25 mg of cortisone acetate. What is the weight of steroid in each tablet?

Molecular weights: cortisone $(C_{21}H_{28}O_5)$ = 360.4; cortisone acetate $(C_{23}H_{30}O_6)$ = 402.5.
Let y be the weight of cortisone in a 25 mg cortisone acetate tablet. By simple proportion:

$$\frac{402.5}{360.4} = \frac{25}{y} \text{ , therefore } y = \frac{25 \times 360.4}{402.5} = 22.39 \text{ mg cortisone.}$$

Example 4.5

Chloramphenicol suspension contains 125 mg chloramphenicol (as palmitate)/5 mL. How many milligrams of chloramphenicol palmitate are required for each 5 mL dose?

Molecular weights: chloramphenicol $(C_{11}H_{12}Cl_2N_2O_5)$ = 323.1; chloramphenicol palmitate $(C_{27}H_{42}Cl_2N_2O_6)$ = 561.5
Expression of the dose of a drug in terms of the base rather than the derivative is common, especially when there are several different derivatives as with chloramphenicol (cinnamate and sodium succinate are also used).
Let y be the actual weight of chloramphenicol palmitate required. Using simple proportion:

$$\frac{323.1}{561.5} = \frac{125}{y} \text{ , therefore } y = \frac{125 \times 561.5}{323.1} = 217.2 \text{ mg}$$

This is rounded to 217 mg per 5 mL dose in answer to this question. However, if the answer were to be used to prepare, for example, 1 L of suspension, then the decimal places would be retained until the calculation was completed and then rounded as appropriate.

Example 4.6

What is the weight of erythromycin lactobionate in a vial containing the equivalent of 1 g of erythromycin for reconstitution?

Molecular weights: erythromycin ($C_{37}H_{67}NO_{13}$) = 733.9; erythromycin lactobionate ($C_{37}H_{67}NO_{13}.C_{12}H_{22}O_{12}$) = 1092.2.

Let y be the weight of erythromycin lactobionate in the vial. By simple proportion:

$$\frac{733.9}{1092.2} = \frac{1}{y}, \text{ therefore } y = \frac{1 \times 1092.2}{733.9} = 1.488 \text{ g.}$$

CALCULATIONS INVOLVING HYDRATES

Example 4.7

Ferrous sulphate is available as anhydrous ferrous sulphate and ferrous sulphate heptahydrate. A pharmacist receives a prescription for 200 mL of Paediatric Ferrous Sulphate Oral Solution and only has anhydrous ferrous sulphate available. How much is required for the medicine?

Molecular weights: anhydrous ferrous sulphate ($FeSO_4$) = 151.9; ferrous sulphate heptahydrate ($FeSO_4.7H_2O$) = 278.0.

The formulation for Paediatric Ferrous Sulphate Solution can be obtained from the *British Pharmacopoeia* (BP) or *British National Formulary* (BNF). It contains ferrous sulphate 60 mg per 5 mL dose. 'Ferrous sulphate' is the heptahydrate.

5 mL of the paediatric solution contains 60 mg of ferrous sulphate. Therefore, 200 mL contains:

$$\frac{60 \times 200}{5} = 2400 \text{ mg} = 2.4 \text{ g.}$$

Let y be the amount of anhydrous ferrous sulphate equivalent to 2.4 g of ferrous sulphate heptahydrate. By simple proportion:

$$\frac{278.0}{151.9} = \frac{2.4}{y}, \text{ therefore } y = \frac{2.4 \times 151.9}{278.0} = 1.311 \text{ g.}$$

1.311 g of anhydrous ferrous sulphate is required.

4

DRUGS IN DIFFERENT FORMS

Example 4.8

Aminophylline is a stable complex of theophylline ($C_7H_8N_4O_2$) and ethylenediamine ($C_2H_8N_2$). It is also a dihydrate. Calculate the weight of aminophylline dihydrate (($C_7H_8N_4O_2)_2.C_2H_8N_2.2H_2O$) and theophylline in a 100 mg tablet of aminophylline. (Answer to 4 significant figures)

Molecular weights: aminophylline (($C_7H_8N_4O_2)_2.C_2H_8N_2$) = 420.5; theophylline = 180.2; aminophylline hydrate = 456.5.
To calculate the amount of aminophylline hydrate, let y be the weight of hydrate. Using simple proportion:

$$\frac{420.5}{456.5} = \frac{100}{y} \text{ , therefore } y = \frac{100 \times 456.5}{420.5} = 108.6 \text{ mg.}$$

To calculate the weight of theophylline, let z be the weight of theophylline. Again using simple proportion:

$$\frac{420.5}{180.2} = \frac{100}{z} \text{ , therefore } z = \frac{100 \times 180.2}{420.5} = 42.85 \text{ mg}$$

Therefore in a 100 mg aminophylline tablet there would be 108.6 mg of aminophylline hydrate which would be equivalent to 42.86 mg of theophylline.

Example 4.9

Codeine Phosphate Oral Solution BP contains 0.5% w/v codeine phosphate BP or an equivalent concentration of codeine phosphate sesquihydrate. Calculate the amount of sesquihydrate required to prepare 100 mL

Molecular weights: codeine phosphate BP is the hemihydrate ($C_{18}H_{21}NO_3.H_3PO_4$ ½H_2O) = 406.4; codeine phosphate sesquihydrate ($C_{18}H_{21}NO_3.H_3PO_4.1$½$H_2O$) = 424.4.
The weight of codeine phosphate must be calculated. 100 mL of a 0.5% solution requires 0.5 g of codeine phosphate.
Let y be the weight of codeine sesquihydrate. Using simple proportion:

$$\frac{406.4}{424.4} = \frac{0.5}{y} \text{ , therefore } y = \frac{0.5 \times 424.4}{406.4} = 0.522 \text{ g}$$

The weight of codeine sesquihydrate to be weighed is 522 mg.

CALCULATIONS WITH LEGAL IMPLICATIONS

The legal classification of a number of drugs is dependent on the amount of drug present in a particular dosage form. With the opioid drugs the concentration is calculated as anhydrous alkaloid. This can determine if the particular medicine is exempt from the normal controlled drug requirements. However, there are other examples.

Example 4.10

Lithium carbonate (Li_2CO_3) is a Prescription Only Medicine (POM) if the dosage to be used contains greater than 5 mg of lithium or the daily dose is to be greater than 15 mg of lithium, otherwise it is a Pharmacy-only medicine (P). What is the legal classification of 200 mg tablets of lithium carbonate?

Molecular weight of lithium carbonate = 73.89.
Let y be the weight of lithium (Atomic weight 6.941).
Using simple proportion:

$$\frac{73.89}{2 \times 6.941} = \frac{200}{y} \text{ , therefore } y = \frac{200 \times 6.941 \times 2}{73.89} = 37.57 \text{ mg.}$$

Therefore, the dose in one tablet is more than seven times the upper limit for the tablets to be considered for P classification. They are, therefore, POM.

Example 4.11

Quinine, as one of its salts, is used in the treatment of malaria. It is normally a POM unless the individual dose is less than the equivalent of 100 mg of quinine base ($C_{20}H_{24}N_2O_2$) and the daily dose is less than the equivalent of 300 mg of quinine. There are commercial 125 mg tablets of quinine sulphate dihydrate (($C_{20}H_{24}N_2O_2)_2.H_2SO_4.2H_2O$). If the maximum dose of these were two daily, could they be sold in a pharmacy?

(Note: the dose suggested is lower than would be used in treating malaria.) Molecular weights: quinine = 324.4; quinine sulphate dihydrate = 782.9.
Let y be the weight of quinine equivalent to the quinine sulphate dihydrate. By simple proportion:

$$\frac{782.9}{2 \times 324.4} = \frac{125}{y} \text{ , therefore } y = \frac{125 \times 324.4 \times 2}{782.9} = 103.6 \text{ mg.}$$

This is more than the legal limit for daily use, so the tablets are a POM medicine.

Example 4.12

A doctor writes a prescription for 100 mL morphine hydrochloride 10 mg/5 mL dose. (a) How much morphine hydrochloride is required? (b) What is the weight of anhydrous morphine base ($C_{17}H_{19}NO_3$) equivalent to the amount of morphine hydrochloride trihydrate

($C_{17}H_{19}NO_3.HCl.3H_2O$) in 100 mL and 5 mL of the solution? (c) What is the legal classification of the mixture?

(Legal status of morphine salts from *Medicines Ethics and Practice*: in liquid preparations, (i) maximum strength 0.2% (calculated as anhydrous morphine base) are classified as CD Inv POM; or (ii) maximum strength 0.02% and maximum dose 3 mg (both calculated as anhydrous morphine base) are classified as CD Inv P, otherwise classified as CD.)

Molecular weights: anhydrous morphine base 285.3; morphine hydrochloride trihydrate 375.8.

(a) 20 doses of morphine hydrochloride are prescribed. Therefore amount required = 20 × 10 = 200 mg morphine hydrochloride.

(b) Let the weight of anhydrous morphine base be y. By simple proportion:

$$\frac{375.8}{285.3} = \frac{200}{y} \text{ , therefore } y = \frac{200 \times 285.3}{375.8} = 151.84 \text{ mg}$$

200 mg of morphine hydrochloride is equivalent to 151.84 mg of anhydrous morphine base in 100 mL. The amount of anhydrous morphine base in 5 mL is:

$$\frac{151.84}{20} = 7.59 \text{ mg.}$$

(c) In order to complete the assessment of the legal status, it is necessary to calculate the percentage strength of the solution. Therefore, 151.84 mg in 100 mL is 0.152% w/v. The mixture has a strength of 0.152% expressed as anhydrous morphine base. The 5 mL dose contains 7.59 mg which is more than 3 mg of anhydrous morphine base, therefore it cannot be CD Inv P. The concentration is less than 0.2% but is greater than 0.02%. Therefore, the mixture is classified as CD Inv POM.

SELF STUDY QUESTIONS

Give all answers to 3 significant figures.

4.1 Calculate the weight of adrenaline (epinephrine) base ($C_9H_{13}NO_3$) in:

(a) 100 μg of adrenaline acid tartrate (epinephrine bitartrate) ($C_9H_{13}NO_3.C_4H_6O_6$)

(b) 100 μg of adrenaline hydrochloride (epinephrine hydrochloride) ($C_9H_{13}NO_3.HCl$)

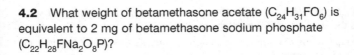

4.2 What weight of betamethasone acetate ($C_{24}H_{31}FO_6$) is equivalent to 2 mg of betamethasone sodium phosphate ($C_{22}H_{28}FNa_2O_8P$)?

4.3 What weight of metronidazole base ($C_6H_9N_3O_3$) is contained in:

(a) 500 mg of metronidazole hydrochloride ($C_6H_9N_3O_3.HCl$)?
(b) 500 mg of metronidazole phosphate ($C_6H_{10}N_3O_6P$)?
(c) 500 mg of metronidazole benzoate ($C_{13}H_{13}N_3O_4$)?

4.4 What weight of clindamycin phosphate ($C_{18}H_{34}ClN_2O_8PS$) is equivalent to 2 g of clindamycin hydrochloride ($C_{18}H_{33}ClN_2O_5S.HCl$)?

4.5 What weight of ergometrine maleate ($C_{19}H_{23}N_3O_2.C_4H_4O_4$) is equivalent to 500 µg of ergometrine tartrate (($C_{19}H_{23}N_3O_2)_2.C_4H_6O_6$)?

4.6 What weight of salt is required to provide 300 mg of chloroquine base ($C_{18}H_{26}ClN_3$)?

(a) Chloroquine hydrochloride ($C_{18}H_{26}ClN_3.2HCl$)
(b) Chloroquine phosphate ($C_{18}H_{26}ClN_3.2H_3PO_4$)
(c) Chloroquine sulphate monohydrate ($C_{18}H_{26}ClN_3.H_2SO_4.H_2O$)

4.7 A tablet contains 2 mg of riboflavin ($C_{17}H_{20}N_4O_6$). What weight of riboflavin sodium phosphate dihydrate ($C_{17}H_{20}N_4NaO_9P.2H_2O$) is equivalent?

4.8 Calculate the amount of salt which is equivalent to 250 mg of quinidine sulphate dihydrate (($C_{20}H_{24}N_2O_2)_2.H_2SO_4.2H_2O$):

(a) Quinidine bisulphate ($C_{20}H_{24}N_2O_2.H_2SO_4$)
(b) Quinidine gluconate ($C_{20}H_{24}N_2O_2.C_6H_{12}O_7$)

4.9 Calculate the weight of warfarin potassium ($C_{19}H_{15}KO_4$) which will provide 5 mg warfarin ($C_{19}H_{16}O_4$).

4.10 Calculate the weight of warfarin sodium ($C_{19}H_{15}NaO_4$) which will provide 5 mg warfarin ($C_{19}H_{16}O_4$).

4.11 Calculate the weight of ester equivalent to 2 mg betamethasone acetate ($C_{24}H_{31}FO_6$):

(a) Betamethasone benzoate ($C_{29}H_{33}FO_6$)
(b) Betamethasone dipropionate ($C_{28}H_{37}FO_7$)
(c) Betamethasone valerate ($C_{27}H_{37}FO_6$)

4.12 Calculate the weight of salt which is equivalent to 600 µg of atropine sulphate monohydrate (($C_{17}H_{23}NO_3)_2.H_2SO_4.H_2O$):

(a) Atropine methobromide ($C_{18}H_{26}BrNO_3$)
(b) Atropine methonitrate ($C_{18}H_{26}N_2O_6$)

4.13 What weight of the following will provide 25 mg hydrocortisone ($C_{21}H_{30}O_5$)?

(a) Hydrocortisone acetate ($C_{23}H_{32}O_6$)
(b) Hydrocortisone cipionate ($C_{29}H_{42}O_6$)
(c) Hydrocortisone valerate ($C_{26}H_{38}O_6$)

4.14 The dose required is 35 µg norethisterone ($C_{20}H_{26}O_2$). What weight of each of the following is required?

(a) Norethisterone acetate ($C_{22}H_{28}O_3$)
(b) Norethisterone enantate ($C_{27}H_{38}O_3$)

4.15 Prochlorperazine mesylate ($C_{20}H_{24}ClN_3S.2CH_3SO_3H$) is available as a mixture containing 5 mg/5 mL:

(a) What concentration of prochlorperazine maleate ($C_{20}H_{24}ClN_3S.2C_4H_4O_4$) is equivalent?
(b) What concentration of prochlorperazine edisilate ($C_{20}H_{24}ClN_3S.C_2H_6O_6S_2$) is equivalent?

4.16 Erythromycin ($C_{37}H_{67}NO_{13}$) capsules contain 250 mg. What weight of ester is required to provide the same amount of erythromycin?

(a) Erythromycin stearate ($C_{37}H_{67}NO_{13}.C_{18}H_{36}O_2$)

(b) Erythromycin ethylsuccinate ($C_{43}H_{75}NO_{16}$)

4.17 Calculate the amount of timolol ($C_{13}H_{24}N_4O_3S$) in 10 mg timolol maleate ($C_{13}H_{24}N_4O_3S.C_4H_4O_4$).

4.18 An injection of testosterone propionate ($C_{22}H_{32}O_3$) contains 50 mg/mL. What is the equivalent concentration of:

(a) Testosterone phenylpropionate ($C_{28}H_{36}O_3$)?
(b) Testosterone isocaproate ($C_{25}H_{38}O_3$)?

4.19 Is 10 mg isosorbide mononitrate ($C_6H_9NO_6$) equivalent to 15 mg isosorbide dinitrate ($C_6H_8N_2O_8$)?

4.20 Calculate the weight of dexamethasone ($C_{22}H_{29}FO_5$) contained in a 2 mL ampoule of dexamethasone sodium phosphate ($C_{22}H_{28}FNa_2O_8P$) 4 mg/mL.

4.21 Calculate the weight of specified element:

(a) Calcium in a 300 mg tablet of fenoprofen calcium dihydrate (($C_{15}H_{13}O_3$)$_2$Ca.2H$_2$O)
(b) Sodium in a 25 mg tablet of diclofenac sodium ($C_{14}H_{10}Cl_2NNaO_2$)
(c) Platinum in a 50 mL ampoule containing 1 mg/mL cisplatin ($H_6Cl_2N_2Pt$)
(d) Gold in a 0.5 mL ampoule of sodium aurothiomalate ($C_4H_3AuNa_2O_4S$) 20 mg/mL
(e) Gold in 3 mg auranofin ($C_{20}H_{34}AuO_9PS$)
(f) Barium in 200 mL of a 5% barium sulphate ($BaSO_4$) suspension
(g) Magnesium in 100 mL of flucloxacillin magnesium octahydrate (($C_{19}H_{16}ClFN_3O_5S$)$_2$Mg.8H$_2$O) 125 mg/5mL
(h) Lithium in 5 mL of 520 mg/5 mL lithium citrate tetrahydrate ($C_6H_5Li_3O_7.4H_2O$)
(i) Iodine in a dose of 50 μg levothyroxine sodium ($C_{15}H_{10}I_4NNaO_4$)

4.22 Calculate the iron content in:

(a) 200 mg ferrous fumarate ($C_4H_2FeO_4$)

(b) 200 mg ferrous gluconate dihydrate ($C_{12}H_{22}FeO_{14}.2H_2O$)

(c) 200 mg ferrous succinate ($C_4H_4FeO_4$)

4.23 Quinine and its salts are P medicines if a single dose does not exceed 100 mg of quinine and the daily dose does not exceed 300 mg of quinine ($C_{20}H_{24}N_2O_2$). Calculate the maximum weight of each salt which will ensure that it is a P medicine, assuming a maximum of three doses daily:

(a) Quinine bisulphate heptahydrate
($C_{20}H_{24}N_2O_2.H_2SO_4.7H_2O$)

(b) Quinine dihydrochloride ($C_{20}H_{24}N_2O_2.2HCl$)

(c) Quinine ethyl carbonate ($C_{23}H_{28}N_2O_4$)

(d) Quinine hydrobromide dihydrate ($C_{20}H_{24}N_2O_2.HBr.2H_2O$)

(e) Quinine hydrochloride dihydrate ($C_{20}H_{24}N_2O_2.HCl.2H_2O$)

(f) Quinine salicylate monohydrate ($C_{20}H_{24}N_2O_2.C_7H_6O_3.H_2O$)

4.24 Liquid preparations of morphine and its salts are controlled as CD Inv P providing that the maximum strength is 0.02% and the maximum dose is 3 mg, both calculated as anhydrous morphine base ($C_{17}H_{19}NO_3$). Calculate the maximum strength (in mg/100 mL) and the maximum single dose of each salt. What would be the volume of the maximum single dose?

(a) Morphine acetate trihydrate ($C_{17}H_{19}NO_3.C_2H_4O_2.3H_2O$)

(b) Morphine hydrochloride trihydrate ($C_{17}H_{19}NO_3.HCl.3H_2O$)

(c) Morphine sulphate pentahydrate
(($C_{17}H_{19}NO_3)_2.H_2SO_4.5H_2O$)

(d) Morphine tartrate trihydrate (($C_{17}H_{19}NO_3)_2.C_4H_6O_6.3H_2O$)

For answers to these questions see page 262

Density

After studying this chapter you will be able to:

- **Define density**
- **Use density of a liquid to convert a weight to volume and vice versa**
- **Use the density measurement in the quality control of syrups**

In Chapter 2 when discussing weights and measures, it was assumed that it is always possible and convenient to measure the volume of a liquid where this is required. However, there are situations where this may not be the case. An example of the latter might be when a very viscous liquid is to be measured. The alternative is to use density in order to convert the volume into a weight.

The density is defined as the mass in grams of 1 millilitre at a specified temperature. Density can be applied to a solid. However, solids are more difficult because they may incorporate air within the particles and there are spaces between the particles in a powder. This means that expressions, such as bulk density, have to be used for expressing the density of solids.

Many official monographs of liquids include a value for the density of the liquid. The *British Pharmacopoeia* (BP) uses the description 'weight per millilitre' and it is for a temperature of 20°C. Since the figures are included as part of the standards for the material, most are quoted as a range rather than a single figure. However, by using a figure at the mid-point of the range, the weight equivalent to the required volume can be calculated.

Example 5.1

A mixture is being prepared which requires the addition of 2 mL of lemon syrup. A suitable measure is not available for this viscous liquid. What weight should be added? (Weight per millilitre = 1.29–1.32 g)

$$\text{Density} = \frac{\text{weight}}{\text{volume}}, \text{ therefore weight} = \text{density} \times \text{volume}$$

$$\text{Density} = \frac{(1.29 + 1.32)}{2} = 1.305 \text{ g/mL}$$

Volume required is 2 mL. Therefore weight = $1.305 \times 2 = 2.61$ g.

Example 5.2

Calamine lotion contains 0.5% v/v liquefied phenol. Liquefied phenol is very caustic and can be difficult to handle. It is decided to weigh the liquefied phenol into the mixture. How much liquefied phenol should be added when producing 50 mL of the lotion? (Weight per millilitre of liquefied phenol = 1.055–1.060 g)

Volume of liquefied phenol is 0.5 mL in 100 mL of lotion.
Therefore in 50 mL of lotion it is 0.25 mL.
Weight required = $0.25 \times (1.055 + 1.060)/2 = 0.264$ g = 264 mg.

Example 5.3

Borax glycerin requires 88% w/w glycerol. In preparing 200 g, 176 g of glycerol is required. What volume would be measured if this were not to be weighed? (Weight per millilitre of glycerol = 1.255–1.260 g)

$$\text{Density} = \frac{\text{weight}}{\text{volume}}, \text{ therefore volume} = \frac{\text{weight}}{\text{density}}$$

Substituting:

$$\text{Volume required} = \frac{176}{1.2575} = 139.96 \text{ mL} = 140 \text{ mL}.$$

Example 5.4

A batch of 1 L of syrup BP has been prepared and is found to weigh 1.295 kg. Does this comply with the requirement for the weight per millilitre of syrup BP?

The BP uses a measure of density to check that Syrup BP is of the required quality. The value should be in the range 1.315–1.333 g/mL. If some of the sugar has not dissolved, the figure will be too low, whilst if water has evaporated the figure will be too high.
Whilst it is not necessary, convert the quantities to units of g and mL.

$$\text{Density} = \text{weight/volume}$$

Substituting:

$$\text{Density} = \frac{1295}{1000} = 1.295 \text{ g/mL}$$

This value is outside the official limits and therefore is not of BP quality.

SELF-STUDY QUESTIONS

Express weights to 2 decimal places, volumes to 1 dp and densities to 3 dp.

5.1 1.3 mL of dill oil is required. What weight should be measured? (Weight per mL 0.895–0.910 g)

5.2 What weight is equivalent to 0.6 mL of chloroform? (Weight per mL 1.474–1.479 g)

5.3 An emulsion requires 75 mL of isopropyl myristate. Given a weight per mL of 0.850–0.855 g, what weight is required?

5.4 Malt extract is being used in a mixture. 12 mL is required and has a weight per mL of 1.489–1.498 g. What weight is required?

5.5 Calculate the weight of eucalyptol to give 5 mL. (Weight per mL 0.922–0.924 g)

5.6 Calculate how much propylene glycol to weigh for a 30 mL quantity. (Weight per mL 1.036–1.038 g)

5.7 Cottonseed oil, 24 g, is required for an emulsion. Calculate the volume. (Weight per mL 0.915–0.920 g)

5.8 When making a suppository base, 24 g liquid macrogol is to be added. What volume will provide this? (Weight per mL 1.120–1.130 g)

5.9 A dilution of glacial acetic acid requires 9 g. What volume should be measured? (Weight per mL 1.048–1.051 g)

5.10 1.5 g cade oil is to be added to an ointment. Calculate the volume to be measured. (Weight per mL 0.970–1.010 g)

5.11 50 g methyl salicylate is required to make a liniment. What is the equivalent volume? (Weight per mL 1.180–1.184 g)

5.12 10% w/w dimeticone is required in 60 g of cream. What volume should be measured? (Weight per mL 0.950–0.965 g)

5.13 12.5% v/w peru balsam is to be incorporated into 50 g of simple ointment. What weight does this represent? (Weight per mL 1.140–1.170 g)

5.14 100 mL of 50% w/v cod liver oil emulsion is being prepared. What volume of oil should be measured? (Weight per mL 0.917–0.924 g)

5.15 An insect repellent preparation will contain 1% w/v dimethyl phthalate. What volume should be measured when making a 1 L batch? (Weight per mL 1.186–1.192 g)

5.16 During the preparation of some 5% v/w lactic acid pessaries, a 75 g batch is being prepared. What weight of lactic acid should be used? (Weight per mL is 1.20 g)

5.17 A 500 mL batch of syrup is found to weigh 681 g. Does this comply with the BP requirement for weight per mL? (Weight per mL is 1.315–1.333 g)

5.18 In order to comply with BP standards, what are the limits of weight of 250 mL of orange syrup? (Weight per mL is 1.315–1.333 g)

5.19 750 mL of lemon syrup has been prepared and found to weigh 953 g. Does this comply with the BP standard? (Weight per mL is 1.315–1.333 g)

5.20 2.5 L of syrup has been prepared and weighs 3315 g. Does this comply with the BP requirements? (Weight per mL is 1.315–1.333 g)

For answers to these questions see page 264

Solubility

After studying this chapter you will be able to

- Express solubility as a percentage and using a '1 part in' description
- Interpret descriptions of solubility
- Calculate the volume of solvent required to prepare a saturated solution
- Determine whether a known quantity of drug will dissolve in the available solvent

When preparing a liquid pharmaceutical product the solubility of all solid ingredients should be checked. This will give useful information on how the product should be prepared. If all ingredients are soluble in the volume of solvent being used a solution can be prepared. However, if one or more of the ingredients is not soluble other formulation techniques may have to be employed to make a solution, or a different type of medicine will have to be produced, such as a suspension or emulsion.

The saturation solubility of a chemical in a solvent is the maximum concentration of a solution which may be prepared at a given temperature. For convenience, this is simply called solubility. Solubilities for medicinal agents in a range of solvents are given in the *British Pharmacopoeia* (BP), *Martindale: The Extra Pharmacopoeia* and a number of other reference sources. Using this information it is often possible to calculate whether a solution can be prepared. It has to be remembered that, as saturation is approached, the rate of solution decreases. Thus it takes longer to make a near-saturated solution than it does a more dilute solution. Thus, most solutions for pharmaceutical use are not saturated

Table 6.1 Phrases used to describe saturation solubility and their approximate meanings (The Pharmaceutical Codex 1994)

Description	Solubility range
Very soluble	less than 1 in 1
Freely soluble	1 in 1 to 1 in 10
Soluble	1 in 10 to 1 in 30
Sparingly soluble	1 in 30 to 1 in 100
Slightly soluble	1 in 100 to 1 in 1000
Very slightly soluble	1 in 1000 to 1 in 10 000
Practically insoluble	1 in greater than 10 000

solutions. Reference to textbooks in pharmaceutics will show that solubility is influenced by a wide range of factors, such as pH and the presence of other materials. In making calculations about solubility in the present context, it is assumed that the solubility given in the official compendium will remain unchanged.

There are two methods of stating solubility in common use. When a material is soluble more than about 1 in 1000, the solubility is usually stated as the number of parts of solvent (by volume) that will dissolve one part (by weight or volume) of the substance. In other situations, words are used to describe the solubility as shown in Table 6.1.

Example 6.1

Potassium chloride is soluble in 2.8 to 3 parts of water.

This means that 1 g of potassium chloride will dissolve in 2.8 to 3 mL of water at a temperature of 20°C (taken as normal room temperature).

Example 6.2

Sodium chloride is soluble 1 in 2.8 of water, 1 in 250 of alcohol and 1 in 10 of glycerol.

This means that 1 g of sodium chloride requires 2.8 mL of water, 250 mL of alcohol or 10 mL of glycerol to dissolve it.

Example 6.3

Diazepam is described as being 'very slightly soluble' in water (which means 1 in 1000 to 1 in 10 000), 'soluble' in alcohol (which means 1 in 10 to 1 in 30) and 'freely soluble' in chloroform (which means 1 in 1 to 1 in 10)

This means that 1 g of diazepam will dissolve in between 1 and 10 mL of chloroform, between 10 and 30 mL of alcohol, but would need 1000 to 10 000 mL of water in which to dissolve, at a temperature of 20°C.

Example 6.4

Express as a percentage the concentration of a saturated solution of atropine in water (solubility 1 in 400 in water).

A saturated solution (y%) is 1 g in 400 mL. To express as a percentage, simple proportion is used, a percentage being parts per hundred. Therefore, let percentage be y:

$$\frac{1 \text{ part}}{400 \text{ parts}} = \frac{y \text{ part}}{100 \text{ parts}}$$

$$y = \frac{1 \times 100}{400} = 0.25\% \text{ w/v}$$

During preparation of medicines, the question is usually, 'Will this amount of material dissolve in the solvent?' or 'How much solvent should be used to dissolve this amount of material?'

Example 6.5

A drug has a solubility of 1 in 80 of water and 1 in 12 of alcohol. Will 200 mg dissolve in 4 mL of water?

1 g of drug will dissolve in 80 mL of water. Let the volume required to dissolve 0.2 g (200 mg) be y:

$$\frac{1}{80} = \frac{0.2}{y}, \text{ therefore } y = \frac{0.2 \times 80}{1} = 16 \text{ mL}$$

Since 16 mL is required to dissolve 200 mg, it will not dissolve in 4 mL. Note: the weight of drug to be dissolved was converted into grams to keep the units consistent throughout the calculation.

Example 6.6

Using the same drug as in Example 6.5, will 5 g dissolve in 60 mL of alcohol?

1 g of drug will dissolve in 12 mL of alcohol. Let the volume of alcohol required to dissolve 5 g be y:

$$\frac{1}{12} = \frac{5}{y}, \text{ therefore } y = \frac{5 \times 12}{1} = 60 \text{ mL}$$

Since the volume of alcohol required to dissolve the 5 g of drug is the same as the volume being used, in theory it will dissolve, but it is a fully saturated solution, so it will be very difficult to achieve in practice.

Example 6.7

Using the same drug as in Example 6.5, will 20 micrograms dissolve in 0.003 mL of water?

1 g of drug will dissolve in 80 mL of water. Let the volume of water required to dissolve 0.00002 g of drug (20 micrograms converted to grams) be y:

$$\frac{1}{80} = \frac{0.00002}{y}, \text{ therefore } y = \frac{0.00002 \times 80}{1} = 0.0016 \text{ mL}.$$

The volume of water required to dissolve the drug is less than the volume available, therefore the drug will dissolve.

Example 6.8

Using the same drug as in Example 6.5, how much water and how much alcohol is required to dissolve 3 g of the drug?

We have established that 1 g of drug will dissolve in 80 mL of water and 12 mL of alcohol. Let y be the amount of water required to dissolve 3 g of drug:

$$\frac{1}{80} = \frac{3}{y}, \text{ therefore } y = \frac{3 \times 80}{1} = 240 \text{ mL water}.$$

Let z be the amount of alcohol required to dissolve 3 g of drug:

$$\frac{1}{12} = \frac{3}{z}, \text{ therefore } z = \frac{3 \times 12}{1} = 36 \text{ mL alcohol}.$$

Therefore, 3 g of the drug will dissolve in 240 mL of water or 36 mL of alcohol.

Example 6.9

The following prescription for eardrops is received. Is it possible to make this as a solution?

Sodium bicarbonate	500 mg
Glycerol	3 mL
Freshly boiled and cooled water to	10 mL
Send	10 mL

Points to note:
Solubility of sodium bicarbonate is 1 in 11 of water.
Glycerol is a viscous liquid which will replace some of the water.
The quantity of water in the eardrops is approximately 6.5 mL.
The question becomes, 'Will 500 mg of sodium bicarbonate dissolve in 6.5 mL of water?'

1 g of sodium bicarbonate will dissolve in 11 mL of water. Let y be the volume of water required to dissolve 0.5 g of sodium bicarbonate:

$$\frac{1}{11} = \frac{0.5}{y}, \text{ therefore } y = \frac{0.5 \times 11}{1} = 5.5 \text{ mL water.}$$

Therefore we require a minimum of 5.5 mL to dissolve the sodium bicarbonate. There is 6.5 mL available, so it will dissolve, but it may be slow as it is approaching saturation.

SELF-STUDY QUESTIONS

6.1 Express the following solubilities as percentages (express to 2 decimal places):

(a) 1 in 30

(b) 1 in 0.3

(c) 1 in 500

(d) 1 in 72

(e) 1 in 4

(f) 1 in 60

(g) 1 in 1

6.2 100 mg will dissolve in what volume of water?

(a) Meprobamate (Solubility 1 in 240)

(b) Propranolol hydrochloride (Solubility 1 in 20)

(c) Methyldopa (Solubility 1 in 100)

(d) Morphine hydrochloride (Solubility 1 in 24)

(e) Paracetamol (Solubility 1 in 70)

(f) Phenobarbital (Solubility 1 in 1000)

(g) Metronidazole (Solubility 1 in 100)

(h) Piperazine phosphate (Solubility 1 in 60)

(i) Salbutamol (Solubility 1 in 70)

(j) Potassium citrate (Solubility 1 in 1)

6.3 How much water is required to dissolve the following?

(a) 1 g of aminophylline (Solubility 1 in 5)

(b) 500 mg of ammonium chloride (Solubility 1 in 2.7)

(c) 100 mg of codeine hydrochloride (Solubility 1 in 20)

(d) 250 mg of apomorphine hydrochloride (Solubility 1 in 50)

(e) 5 g of aspirin (Solubility 1 in 300)

(f) 50 mg of lithium carbonate (Solubility 1 in 100)

(g) 25 g of ferrous gluconate (Solubility 1 in 10)

(h) 5 mg of atropine (Solubility 1 in 400)
(i) 50 mg of morphine sulphate (Solubility 1 in 21)
(j) 40 mg of hydralazine hydrochloride (Solubility 1 in 25)

6.4 How much of each drug will dissolve in 200 mL of water? (Answer to 2 decimal places)

(a) Piperazine phosphate (Solubility 1 in 60)
(b) Quinine hydrochloride (Solubility 1 in 23)
(c) Atropine (Solubility 1 in 400)
(d) Ferrous gluconate (Solubility 1 in 10)
(e) Paracetamol (Solubility 1 in 70)
(f) Codeine sulphate (Solubility 1 in 30)
(g) Morphine sulphate (Solubility 1 in 21)
(h) Phenobarbital (Solubility 1 in 1000)
(i) Aminophylline (Solubility 1 in 5)
(j) Propranolol hydrochloride (Solubility 1 in 20)

6.5 How much of each drug will dissolve in 20 mL of water? If 200 mg is to be dispensed, will it dissolve in 20 mL of water?

(a) Theophylline (Solubility 1 in 120)
(b) Isoniazid (Solubility 1 in 8)
(c) Lithium carbonate (Solubility 1 in 100)
(d) Quinine sulphate (Solubility 1 in 810)
(e) Lidocaine hydrochloride (lignocaine hydrochloride) (Solubility 1 in 0.7)
(f) Potassium citrate (Solubility 1 in 1)
(g) Meprobamate (Solubility 1 in 240)
(h) Metronidazole (Solubility 1 in 100)
(i) Morphine hydrochloride (Solubility 1 in 24)

6.6 Convert each solubility to a percentage (to 2 decimal places):

(a) 1 in 25   **(e)** 1 in 240
(b) 1 in 810   **(f)** 1 in 2.7
(c) 1 in 0.7   **(g)** 1 in 50
(d) 1 in 8   **(h)** 1 in 21

6.7 Express 300 mg in 30 mL as a 1 in . . . solution.

6.8 300 mg is to be dispensed, will it dissolve in 30 mL of water?

(a) Quinine hydrobromide (Solubility 1 in 55)
(b) Apomorphine hydrochloride (Solubility 1 in 50)
(c) Hydralazine hydrochloride (Solubility 1 in 25)
(d) Cimetidine (Solubility 1 in 200)
(e) Caffeine (Solubility 1 in 60)
(f) Ammonium chloride (Solubility 1 in 2.7)
(g) Aspirin (Solubility 1 in 300)

6.9 Calculate the amount of water required to dissolve the following:

(a) 250 mg of caffeine (Solubility 1 in 60)
(b) 2.5 g of ergometrine maleate (Solubility 1 in 40)
(c) 2.5 g of ergotamine tartrate (Solubility 1 in 500)
(d) 1 kg of isoniazid (Solubility 1 in 8)
(e) 400 mg of codeine sulphate (Solubility 1 in 30)
(f) 400 mg of codeine (Solubility 1 in 120)
(g) 15 mg of hydrocortisone sodium succinate (Solubility 1 in 3)
(h) 1.5 g of lidocaine hydrochloride (lignocaine hydrochloride) (Solubility 1 in 0.7)
(i) 300 mg of cimetidine (Solubility 1 in 200)

6.10 How much of each drug will dissolve in 10 mL of water? If 500 mg is to be dispensed, will each dissolve in 50 mL of water?

(a) Ergometrine maleate (Solubility 1 in 40)
(b) Ergotamine tartrate (Solubility 1 in 500)
(c) Codeine hydrochloride (Solubility 1 in 20)
(d) Codeine (Solubility 1 in 120)

6.11 How much water is required to dissolve 2.0 g of each of the following salts? Which one is most soluble in water?

(a) Quinine hydrobromide (Solubility 1 in 55)

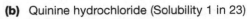

(b) Quinine hydrochloride (Solubility 1 in 23)

(c) Quinine sulphate (Solubility 1 in 810)

For answers to these questions see page 265

Master formulae

After studying this chapter you will be able to:

- Distinguish between formulae which specify quantities of all ingredients and formulae to be made to a final weight or volume
- Scale formulae to larger or smaller quantities using either proportion calculations or a scaling factor
- Handle formulae written with quantities, parts and percentages
- Calculate for additional materials in suspensions and emulsions

INTRODUCTION

In extemporaneous dispensing the names and quantities of the ingredients are provided on the prescription or have to be obtained from a recognized reference source. There are many reference sources used. The most common are the various national Pharmacopoeias and *Martindale—The Extra Pharmacopoeia*. The contents of these reference sources have changed over the years, with the focus moving towards pre-manufactured medicines. Therefore, there are many more formulae in earlier editions than in more recent editions. Where a prescription for an extemporaneous medicine is from an official compendium it will be named with letters such as BP, BPC, BNF added. This indicates the source which should be consulted. When searching back through different editions, the most recent one containing the formula should be used.

Whether the medicine is defined on the prescription or through an official compendium, the list of ingredients and quantities is the 'master formula' for that medicine.

Traditionally, they were referred to as the 'recipe', hence the use of the symbol ℞, which is an abbreviation for 'recipe', at the start of a prescription. As with any recipe, they give the information about the ingredients and quantities, but the method of preparation is not included—and is beyond the scope of this book. The 'master formula' may be written for different final quantities. Thus it could be written for an individual dose (e.g. 5 mL), for the quantity requested (e.g. 50 g), for a nominal quantity (e.g. 100 g or 1000 mL) or some other less obvious quantity. Unless the master formula is written for the quantity to be provided, the master formula quantities will have to be scaled to produce the required quantity. In some situations, for example when preparing ointments and creams, it is necessary to prepare more than is to be dispensed due to losses during production. More information about these can be obtained in *Pharmaceutical Practice*, 3rd edition. Scaling of the master formula is carried out in one of two, interrelated, ways. One is to use simple proportion, the other derives a 'multiplying factor'. The latter is the ratio of the required quantity divided by the formula quantity. The examples in this chapter will illustrate these processes.

There are two other important aspects of the master formula which must be dealt with before considering individual examples. A master formula can be written in a form where the quantity of each ingredient is specified (see Example 7.1), or where one ingredient is used to make the quantity up to the required weight or volume (see Example 7.2). In the latter case, the quantity value for the final ingredient is preceded by the word 'to', or 'ad' in some older sources. Obviously the calculations involved are different in the two cases, as will be demonstrated by the examples which follow. In Chapter 2 there was consideration of different ways in which quantities can be expressed. All these can be found in master formulae. When reading formulae it is important to determine the ways in which quantities are expressed and handle them appropriately. This is especially true when more than one way (e.g. volume and percentage) is used in the same master formula, since different methods of processing the scaling may be required.

FORMULAE WHERE WEIGHTS AND VOLUMES ARE USED

Example 7.1

Calculate the quantities to prepare the following product: 50 g Compound Benzoic Acid Ointment BPC

The *British Pharmaceutical Codex* (last published in 1979) gives the master formula as:

Ingredient	Quantity
Benzoic acid	6 g
Salicylic acid	3 g
Emulsifying ointment	91 g

All quantities in the master formula are given in grams and they add up to 100 g. This indicates that the final product will be made by weight and that there will be no final adjustment to weight.

The master formula is for 100 g, but the request is for 50 g, therefore it will be necessary to scale the quantities. This can be achieved either by using simple proportion or by calculating and applying a scaling factor.

(a) By simple proportion

Benzoic acid   6 g

Let y be the amount of benzoic acid required. By simple proportion:

$$\frac{6}{100} = \frac{y}{50} \text{ , therefore } y = \frac{6 \times 50}{100} = 3 \text{ g.}$$

Salicylic acid   3 g

Let z be the amount of salicylic acid required. By simple proportion:

$$\frac{3}{100} = \frac{z}{50} \text{ , therefore } z = \frac{3 \times 50}{100} = 1.5 \text{ g.}$$

Emulsifying ointment   91 g

Let w be the amount of emulsifying ointment required. By simple proportion:

$$\frac{91}{100} = \frac{w}{50} \text{ , therefore } w = \frac{91 \times 50}{100} = 45.5 \text{ g.}$$

From these calculations we can write the master formula and the scaled (i.e. required) quantities:

Ingredient	Quantity	Scaled quantity
Benzoic acid	6 g	3 g
Salicylic acid	3 g	1.5 g
Emulsifying ointment	91 g	45.5 g

Note: It is easy to double-check the individual quantities because they should add up to 50 g. They do.

(b) Using a scaling factor

The scaling factor is simply the ratio of the required quantity to the formula quantity. In this example the scaling factor is:

$$\frac{50}{100} = 0.5.$$

The scaling factor is then used to multiply each of the quantities in the master formula.

Ingredient	Quantity	Scaling	Scaled quantity
Benzoic acid	6 g	6×0.5 g	3 g
Salicylic acid	3 g	3×0.5 g	1.5 g
Emulsifying ointment	91 g	91×0.5 g	45.5 g

Again it can be confirmed that the quantities add up to 50 g.

Example 7.2

Prepare 100 mL of Chloroform Emulsion BPC

Ingredient	Quantity
Chloroform	50 mL
Quillaia liquid extract	1 mL
Tragacanth mucilage	50 mL
Water	to 1000 mL

Water is being used as the vehicle in this emulsion and a sufficient quantity is to be added to make the required volume. The master formula is for 1000 mL, the required amount is 100 mL, therefore scaling will be required. This can be carried out using either proportion or a scaling factor. The scaling factor will be:

$$\frac{100}{1000} = 0.1.$$

Ingredient	Quantity	By proportion	By scaling factor	Required
Chloroform	50 mL	$\dfrac{50 \times 100}{1000}$	50×0.1	5 mL
Quillaia liquid extract	1 mL	$\dfrac{1 \times 100}{1000}$	1×0.1	0.1 mL
Tragacanth mucilage	50 mL	$\dfrac{50 \times 100}{1000}$	50×0.1	5 mL
Water	to 1000 mL	–	–	to 100 mL

There is no calculation for the quantity of water because we do not need to know how much to add. However, in this example, where all the ingredients are measured as volumes, it is possible to calculate how much water is required.

Required water for 1000 mL = 1000 − (50 + 1 + 50) = 899 mL

From this figure we could calculate the amount required in the final emulsion.

Ingredient	Quantity	By proportion	By scaling factor	Required
Water	899 mL	$\dfrac{899 \times 100}{1000}$	899×0.1	89.9 mL

Without carrying out the calculation for water, it would not be possible to check that the total volume of liquids being added came to 100 mL. It can now be seen that they add up correctly.

Example 7.3

℞

200 mL of Ammonium Chloride Mixture BPC

The formula can be found in a variety of reference books, such as *Martindale—The Extra Pharmacopoeia* in addition to the *Pharmaceutical Codex*. When using 'Martindale' as the source the master formula gives quantities sufficient for 10 mL.

The prescription is for 200 mL and is a mixture of both solids and liquids, using water as the vehicle. It may be calculated using proportion or by multiplying by a scaling factor which is 200/10 = 20.

Ingredient	Formula quantity	Proportion	By factor	Quantity
Ammonium chloride	1 g	$\dfrac{1 \times 200}{10}$	1×20	20 g
Aromatic solution of ammonia	0.5 mL	$\dfrac{0.5 \times 200}{10}$	0.5×20	10 mL
Liquorice liquid extract	1 mL	$\dfrac{1 \times 200}{10}$	1×20	20 mL
Water	to 10 mL	–	–	to 200 mL

As with Example 7.2 there is no calculation for the amount of water because it is being used to make up to final volume. In this case, because we have a mixture of both solids and liquids, it is not possible to calculate the exact quantity of water which is required. However, it is always good practice to have an idea of what the approximate quantity will be. The liquid ingredients of the preparation, other than the water, add up to 30 mL and there is 20 g of ammonium chloride. The volume of water required will therefore be in the region of 150 mL.

In most formulae where a combination of weights and volumes is required the formula will indicate that the preparation is to be made up to the required weight or volume with the designated vehicle. However, occasionally, as can be seen in the next example, a combination of weights and volumes is used and it is not possible to indicate what the exact final weight or volume of the preparation will be. In these instances an excess quantity is normally calculated for and the required amount measured.

Example 7.4
Calculate the quantities required to produce 300 mL Turpentine Liniment BP 1988.

Ingredient	Master formula
Soft soap	75 g
Camphor	50 g
Turpentine oil	650 mL
Water	225 mL

When the total number of units is added up for this formula it comes to 1000. However, because it is a combination of solids and liquids, it cannot be predicted if it will produce 1000 mL. It is known from experience that it will produce approximately 890 mL. The prescription is for 300 mL so calculate for 340 units which will provide slightly more than 300 mL. The required amount can then be measured. The value of '340' is used in either proportion or scaling factor calculation methods.

$$\text{Scaling factor} = 340/1000 = 0.34.$$

Ingredient	Master quantity	Proportion	By factor	Quantity for 340 units
Soft soap	75 g	$\frac{75 \times 340}{1000}$	75×0.34	25.5 g
Camphor	50 g	$\frac{50 \times 340}{1000}$	50×0.34	17 g
Turpentine oil	650 mL	$\frac{650 \times 340}{1000}$	650×0.34	221 mL
Water	225 mL	$\frac{225 \times 340}{1000}$	225×0.34	76.5 mL

CALCULATIONS INVOLVING PARTS

In the following example the quantities are expressed as parts of the whole. The number of parts is added up and the quantity of each ingredient calculated by proportion or multiplying factor, to provide the correct amounts.

Example 7.5
℞

Methyl salicylate	1 part
Arachis oil	to 4 parts
Send 200 mL	

Because the prescription is written as 'to' 4 parts, there are 3 parts of arachis oil. As previously, the quantities can be calculated using either proportion or scaling factor. The scaling factor can be calculated as $200/4 = 50$.

Ingredient	Formula	Proportion	By scaling	Quantity
Methyl salicylate	1 part	$\dfrac{1 \times 200}{4}$	1×50	50 mL
Arachis oil	3 parts	$\dfrac{3 \times 200}{4}$	3×50	150 mL

It is obvious that the quantities add up to 200 mL. Also, by observation, the ratios are as expected from the prescription.

Example 7.6
30 g of the following product is to be prepared:

Ingredient	Quantity
Zinc oxide	12.5 parts
Calamine	15 parts
Hydrous wool fat	25 parts
White soft paraffin	47.5 parts

The total number of parts adds up to 100. The scaling factor is $30/100 = 0.3$.

Ingredient	Quantity	Proportion	Scaling	Quantity for 30 g
Zinc oxide	12.5 parts	$\dfrac{12.5 \times 30}{100}$	12.5×0.3	3.75 g
Calamine	15 parts	$\dfrac{15 \times 30}{100}$	15×0.3	4.5 g
Hydrous wool fat	25 parts	$\dfrac{25 \times 30}{100}$	25×0.3	7.5 g
White soft paraffin	47.5 parts	$\dfrac{47.5 \times 30}{100}$	47.5×0.3	14.25 g

The quantities add up to 30 g. It is also possible to notice that the calamine at 15 parts is slightly more than the zinc oxide at 12.5 parts and that the hydrous wool fat, at 25 parts, is exactly double the zinc oxide at 12.5 parts.

Example 7.7

℞

Zinc sulphate	1 part
Amaranth solution	1 part
Water	to 100 parts
Send 250 mL	

This is a mixture of solids and liquids, to be made up to 100 parts.
The scaling factor will be 250/100 = 2.5.

Ingredient	Quantity	Proportion	By factor	Required quantity
Zinc sulphate	1 part	$\dfrac{1 \times 250}{100}$	1×2.5	2.5 g
Amaranth solution	1 part	$\dfrac{1 \times 250}{100}$	1×2.5	2.5 mL
Water	to 100 parts	–	–	to 250 mL

There are some situations when extra care is necessary in
reading the prescription.

Example 7.8

Two products are to be dispensed:

Betnovate® cream	1 part
Aqueous cream	to 4 parts
Prepare 50 g	

Haelan® ointment	1 part
White soft paraffin	4 parts
Prepare 50 g	

At first glance these calculations look similar but the quantities
required for each are different. In the Betnovate prescription the total
number of parts is 4, i.e. 1 part of Betnovate and 3 parts of aqueous
cream to produce a total of 4 parts. However, in the Haelan
prescription the total number of parts is 5, i.e. 1 part of Haelan
ointment and 4 parts of white soft paraffin.
The quantities required for the prescriptions are as follows:

Betnovate cream	12.5 g
Aqueous cream	37.5 g
And for the second one:	
Haelan ointment	10 g
White soft paraffin	40 g

CALCULATIONS INVOLVING PERCENTAGES

There should be no problems in calculating from percentages, but many students make mistakes, most often because they apply the scaling or proportion to the percentage. This is incorrect, since the percentage is an expression based on the final quantity produced. A simple way around the problem is to convert the percentage into a weight or volume as the first step of the calculation. There is then no further problem, providing the correct conventions are applied in the process.

These conventions apply when dealing with formulae which include percentages:

- A solid in a formula where the final quantity is stated as a weight is calculated as weight in weight (w/w).
- A solid in a formula where the final quantity is stated as a volume is calculated as weight in volume (w/v).
- A liquid in a formula where the final quantity is stated as a volume is calculated as volume in volume (v/v).
- A liquid in a formula where the final quantity is stated as a weight is calculated as weight in weight (w/w).

Example 7.9
Prepare 250 g of the following ointment:

Ingredient	Formula
Sulphur	2%
Salicylic acid	1%
White soft paraffin	to 10 g

The ingredients specified as percentages are solids and the final product is given as a weight. Therefore, using the convention, the percentages are treated as weight in weight (w/w).
The master formula is for a total of 10 g. The scaling factor is:

$$\frac{250}{10} = 25.$$

The first step is to convert the percentages into quantities—weights in this example. Remember, do not multiply the percentage figure. This always remains the same no matter how much is being prepared.

Ingredient	Formula	Converted	Proportion	Scaled	Quantity for 250 g
Sulphur	2%	0.2 g	$\dfrac{0.2 \times 250}{10}$	0.2×25	5 g
Salicylic acid	1%	0.1 g	$\dfrac{0.1 \times 250}{10}$	0.1×25	2.5 g
White soft paraffin	to 10 g	to 10 g	–	–	242.5 g

Example 7.10
℞

Sulfacetamide sodium	3%
Water for injections	to 100 mL
Send 10 mL	

In this preparation we have a solid given as a percentage to be dissolved in a liquid to give a final volume. Therefore the convention is that this is a weight in volume percentage (w/v).
Convert the percentage into an actual quantity:

3% w/v is 3 g in 100 mL.
The scaling factor is 10/100 = 0.1.

Ingredient	Quantity	Converted	Proportion	Scaling	Quantity for 10 mL
Sulfacetamide sodium	3%	3 g	$\dfrac{3 \times 10}{100}$	3×0.1	0.3 g
Water	to 100 mL	to 100 mL	–	–	to 10 mL

Example 7.11
℞

Hydrogen peroxide solution (6%)	25%
Water	to 100 mL
Send 20 mL of eardrops	

The percentage here is a liquid and the final product is also a liquid, so this is treated as a volume in volume (v/v) solution.
Convert the percentage into a volume:

25% v/v in 100 mL is 25 mL.
Scaling factor = 20/100 = 0.2.

Ingredient	Quantity	Converted	Proportion	Scaling	Quantity
Hydrogen peroxide solution (6%)	25%	25 mL	$\dfrac{25 \times 20}{100}$	25×0.2	5.0 mL
Water	to 100 mL	to 100 mL	–	–	to 20 mL

Example 7.12

℞

Coal tar solution	3%
Zinc oxide	2.5 g
Yellow soft paraffin	to 50 g
Send 60 g	

In this example a liquid ingredient, the coal tar solution, is stated as a percentage and a weight in grams of final product is requested. The convention requires a percentage weight in weight (w/w). Note also that the total product is given as 50 g. The coal tar solution is a weight (3 g in 100 g) and the zinc oxide is also a weight but in a different quantity (2.5 g in 50 g). Care is required to ensure that the correct answer is arrived at without confusing the two different denominators of proportion. The first step is to convert the percentage into a finite weight. Convert the percentage:

$$\frac{3 \times 50}{100} = 1.5 \text{ g in 50 g ointment}$$

It is also possible to calculate the amount of yellow soft paraffin which is required, because it is weight in weight. It is
50 − (1.5 + 2.5) = 46 g.
The quantity to be made is 60 g so the scaling factor is 60/50 = 1.2.

Ingredient	Quantity	Converted	Proportion	Scaling	Quantity for 60 g
Coal tar solution	3%	1.5 g	$\frac{1.5 \times 60}{50}$	1.5 × 1.2	1.8 g
Zinc oxide	2.5 g	2.5 g	$\frac{2.5 \times 60}{50}$	2.5 × 1.2	3 g
Yellow soft paraffin	to 50 g	46 g	$\frac{46 \times 60}{50}$	46 × 1.2	55.2 g

Check that the weights add up to 60 g.

Example 7.13

Sometimes, prescriptions are written to give 100 parts. These can be treated as percentages. This is an example:

℞

Sodium bicarbonate	2
Borax	2
Glycerol	10
Water	to 100
Send 150 mL	

This is written as parts, but because the total number of parts is 100, each figure is actually a percentage. Therefore the calculations are simple using proportion or the scaling factor. The scaling factor is $150/100 = 1.5$.

Ingredient	Quantity	Proportion	Scaling	Final quantity
Sodium bicarbonate	2	$\dfrac{2 \times 150}{100}$	2×1.5	3 g
Borax	2	$\dfrac{2 \times 150}{100}$	2×1.5	3 g
Glycerol	10	$\dfrac{10 \times 150}{100}$	10×1.5	15 mL
Water	to 100	–	–	to 150 mL

Since there is a mixture of solids and liquids, the amount of water to add cannot be calculated. However, it may be noted that there are five times as many parts of glycerol as there of the two solids, and the volume of glycerol is numerically five times the weight of the solids.

Example 7.14
When dealing with preparations where ingredients are expressed as a percentage concentration, it is important to check if the standard conventions apply because there are some situations where they do not apply. Two examples are given below.

(a) Syrup BP is a liquid—a solution of sucrose and water. If the normal convention applied it would be w/v, i.e. a certain weight of sucrose in a final volume of syrup. However, in the BP formula the concentration of sucrose is quoted as w/w. Therefore Syrup BP is:

Sucrose   66.7% w/w
Water   to 100%

This means that when preparing Syrup BP the appropriate weight of sucrose is weighed out and water is added to the required weight, not volume.

Suppose there is a request to prepare 1 L of syrup. Because of the density of syrup, making 1 kg will not produce 1 L. From Chapter 5 you should be able to work out what volume it will produce. Let us now assume that the request is for 1000 g. This may be calculated by proportion or scaling factor. The scaling factor is $1000/100 = 10$.

Ingredient	Quantity	Proportion	Scaling	Final quantity
Sucrose	66.7% (w/w)	$\dfrac{66.7 \times 1000}{100}$	66.7×10	667 g
Water	33.3% (w/w)	$\dfrac{33.3 \times 1000}{100}$	33.3×10	333 g

In practice, rather than adding a finite quantity, water is added to bring up to final weight at the end, because a heating process is used which can cause some water to evaporate during preparation.

(b) A gas in a solution is always calculated as w/w, unless specified otherwise. Formaldehyde Solution BP is a solution of 34–38% w/w formaldehyde in water. Hydrogen peroxide is also a gas dissolved in water. However, in this case both w/w and w/v units are used in the official compendia. For example, Hydrogen Peroxide Solution (30%) BP is described as being 29–31% w/w, whilst Hydrogen Peroxide Solution (6%) BP is described as being 5–7% w/v. Hydrogen peroxide solutions are open to confusion because of this and also because they may be described in terms of 'volumes' as described in Chapter 2.

FORMULAE WHERE ADDITIONAL MATERIALS ARE REQUIRED

There are a number of situations where, in order to produce a stable medicine, additional materials, not included in the prescription, have to be added. A discussion of the reasons for these additions is beyond the scope of this book, but further information is included in appropriate chapters of the 3rd edition of *Pharmaceutical Practice*. The need to add diluents during trituration is dealt with in Chapter 9 and the use of suppository bases and displacement values are covered in Chapter 10 of this book.

Example 7.15
℞

Chalk	120 mg
Syrup	0.5 mL
Concentrated cinnamon water	0.02 mL
Double strength chloroform water	2.5 mL
Water	to 5 mL

Send 150 mL

This suspension has an indiffusible solid, chalk, and so requires a suspending agent. These suspending agents are added as a percentage of the final volume. The two common materials used are Tragacanth Powder at 0.2% w/v and Compound Tragacanth Powder at 2.0% w/v. The BP uses Tragacanth Powder for a very similar mixture, and so it is used in this case. The master formula is modified to the following and the calculations carried out as before. The scaling factor is 150/5 = 30.

Ingredient	Quantity	Converted	Proportion	Scaling	Quantity
Chalk	120 mg	0.120 g	$\dfrac{0.120 \times 150}{5}$	0.120×30	3.6 g
Syrup	0.5 mL	0.5 mL	$\dfrac{0.5 \times 150}{5}$	0.5×30	15 mL
Concentrated cinnamon water	0.02 mL	0.02 mL	$\dfrac{0.02 \times 150}{5}$	0.02×30	0.6 mL
Double strength chloroform water	2.5 mL	2.5 mL	$\dfrac{2.5 \times 150}{5}$	2.5×30	75 mL
Tragacanth powder	0.2%	10 mg	$\dfrac{10 \times 150}{5}$	10×30	300 mg
Water	to 5 mL	to 5 mL	–	–	to 150 mL

Example 7.16

℞

Menthol	2 g
Eucalyptus oil	10 mL
Water	to 100 mL
Make 100 mL	

This inhalation requires an adsorbent for the oils so that they can be dispersed through the water. Light magnesium carbonate is used for this at a rate of about 1 g of light magnesium carbonate per 2 mL or 2 g of oily material. In this case, whilst the menthol is a solid it dissolves in the eucalyptus oil to produce a liquid. Therefore the amount of light magnesium carbonate required is (10 + 2)/2 = 6 g. A small excess will provide a larger surface area for adsorption, so 7 g can be used. The formula becomes:

Menthol	2 g
Eucalyptus oil	10 mL
Light magnesium carbonate	7 g
Water	to 100 mL

These are the actual quantities required, so no further calculation is necessary.

Emulsions

Emulsions are dispersions of oil in water, or vice versa, and require the addition of an emulsifying agent. In extemporaneous dispensing this is usually acacia powder, the actual amount required depending on the nature of the oil. During preparation a 'primary emulsion' is first formed, using

Table 7.1   Ratios used for primary emulsions

Type of oil	Examples	Oil	Water	Acacia
Fixed	Almond, arachis, cod liver, castor	4	2	1
Mineral (hydrocarbon)	Liquid paraffin	3	2	1
Volatile	Turpentine, cinnamon, peppermint	2	2	1
Oleo-resin	Male fern extract	1	2	1

optimum proportions of oil, water and acacia. The recommended proportions are shown in Table 7.1. There are, therefore, two stages to the calculation from a master formula for an emulsion; the overall composition and the composition of the primary emulsion.

Example 7.17

Calculate the quantities for a primary emulsion for the following:

℞

Cod liver oil	30 mL
Water	to 100 mL
Send 200 mL	

First calculate the total quantities required for the emulsion using proportion or scaling. Scaling factor is 200/100 = 2.

Ingredient	Quantity	Proportion	Scaling	Required quantity
Cod liver oil	30 mL	$\dfrac{30 \times 200}{100}$	30×2	60 mL
Water	to 100 mL	–	–	to 200 mL

Primary emulsion quantities

Cod liver oil is a fixed oil, therefore the primary emulsion proportions are 4 : 2 : 1. Hence:

Cod liver oil	60 mL	(4 parts)
Water	30 mL	(2 parts)
Powdered acacia gum	15 g	(1 part)

More water is added later to give the 200 mL required.

An additional complication with emulsions arises when the proportion of oil in the emulsion is lower than about 20%, because this leads to instability. In such situations the

formulation must be modified, by adding an inert oil to bring
the proportion up to at least 20% v/v. Fixed oils such as
arachis, sesame, cottonseed or maize oil can be used.

Example 7.18
℞

Send 50 mL calciferol solution containing 0.15 mL per 5 mL dose.
The percentage of calciferol in each dose is 3%. Calciferol is an oil,
but the oil content must be made up to at least 20% to produce a
stable emulsion. In this case cottonseed oil will be used as the
bulking oil.
Since 20% of 5 mL = 1 mL, the volume of cottonseed oil required is
1 – 0.15 = 0.85 mL. The master formula and calculations become:

Ingredient	Quantity	Proportion	Scaling	Final quantity
Calciferol solution	0.15 mL	$\dfrac{0.15 \times 50}{5}$	0.15×10	1.5 mL
Cottonseed oil	0.85 mL	$\dfrac{0.85 \times 50}{5}$	0.85×10	8.5 mL
Water	to 5 mL	–	–	to 50 mL

Formula for primary emulsion (for 50 mL):

Calciferol solution	1.5 mL	(together are 4 parts)
Cottonseed oil	8.5 mL	
Water	5 mL	(2 parts)
Acacia	2.5 g	(1 part)

SELF-STUDY QUESTIONS

Calculate the quantities of ingredients required for the following products:

7.1 **(a)** Belladonna tincture 40 mL
Benzoic acid solution 20 mL
Glycerol 100 mL
Syrup 200 mL
Water to 1000 mL
Send 50 mL

(b) Belladonna tincture 40 mL
Benzoic acid solution 20 mL
Glycerol 100 mL
Syrup 200 mL
Water to 1000 mL
Send 120 mL

(c) Belladonna tincture 4 mL
Benzoic acid solution 2 mL
Glycerol 10 mL
Syrup 20 mL
Water to 100 mL
Send 60 mL

7.2 **(a)** Starch 350 g
Zinc oxide 300 g
Olive oil 200 g
Wool fat 150 g
Send 30 g

(b) Hydrocortisone 10 g
Oxytetracycline 30 g
Wool fat 100 g
White soft paraffin 860 g
Send 50 g

(c) White beeswax 200 mg
Hard paraffin 300 mg
Cetostearyl alcohol 0.5 g

	Soft paraffin	9 g
	Send 75 g	
(d)	Starch	35 g
	Zinc oxide	30 g
	Olive oil	20 g
	Wool fat	15 g
	Send 30 g	
(e)	Hydrocortisone	1 g
	Oxytetracycline	3 g
	Wool fat	10 g
	White soft paraffin	86 g
	Send 60 g	
(f)	Starch	3.5 g
	Zinc oxide	3 g
	Olive oil	2 g
	Wool fat	1.5 g
	Send 75 g	
(g)	Wool alcohols	6 g
	Soft paraffin	10 g
	Hard paraffin	24 g
	Liquid paraffin	60 g
	Send 60 g	
(h)	Hydrocortisone	1 g
	Oxytetracycline	3 g
	Wool fat	10 g
	White soft paraffin	86 g
	Send 30 g	
(i)	White beeswax	20 g
	Hard paraffin	30 g
	Cetostearyl alcohol	50 g
	Soft paraffin	900 g
	Send 150 g	
(j)	Wool alcohols	600 mg
	Soft paraffin	1 g
	Hard paraffin	2.4 g
	Liquid paraffin	6 g
	Send 75 g	

7.3 **(a)** Light magnesium carbonate — 3 g
Sodium bicarbonate — 5 g
Aromatic cardamom tincture — 3 mL
Chloroform water, double strength — 50 mL
Water — to 100 mL
Send 60 mL

(b) Magnesium sulphate — 400 g
Light magnesium carbonate — 50 g
Concentrated peppermint water — 25 g
Chloroform water, double strength — 300 mL
Water — to 1000 mL
Send 150 mL

(c) Light magnesium carbonate — 3 g
Sodium bicarbonate — 5 g
Aromatic cardamom tincture — 3 mL
Chloroform water, double strength — 50 mL
Water — to 100 mL
Send 120 mL

(d) Magnesium sulphate — 4 g
Light magnesium carbonate — 0.5 g
Concentrated peppermint water — 250 mg
Chloroform water, double strength — 3 mL
Water — to 10 mL
Send 75 mL

(e) Magnesium trisilicate — 5 g
Light magnesium carbonate — 7.5 g
Sodium bicarbonate — 2.5 g
Chloroform water, double strength — 50 mL
Water — to 100 mL
Send 120 mL

7.4 **(a)** Resorcinol — 5 parts
Precipitated sulphur — 10 parts
Zinc oxide — 40 parts
Emulsifying ointment — 45 parts
Send 30 g

(b) Starch — 35 parts
Zinc oxide — 40 parts

| Olive oil | 10 parts |
| Wool fat | 15 parts |

Send 30 g

(c)
Wool fat	5 parts
Hard paraffin	2.5 parts
Cetostearyl alcohol	7.5 parts
Soft paraffin	85 parts

Send 60 g

(d)
Resorcinol	5 parts
Precipitated sulphur	10 parts
Zinc oxide	40 parts
Emulsifying ointment	45 parts

Send 120 g

(e)
Resorcinol	1 part
Precipitated sulphur	2 parts
Zinc oxide	8 parts
Emulsifying ointment	9 parts

Send 30 g

(f)
Wool fat	5 parts
Hard paraffin	2.5 parts
Cetostearyl alcohol	7.5 parts
Soft paraffin	85 parts

Send 120 g

(g)
White beeswax	20 parts
Hard paraffin	30 parts
Cetostearyl alcohol	50 parts
Soft paraffin	900 parts

Send 60 g

(h)
Hard paraffin	4 parts
Soft paraffin	21 parts
Liquid paraffin	5 parts

Send 100 g

(i)
White beeswax	2 parts
Hard paraffin	3 parts
Cetostearyl alcohol	5 parts
Soft paraffin	90 parts

Send 120 g

(j) Ichthammol   5 parts
    Cetostearyl alcohol   3 parts
    Wool fat   10 parts
    Zinc cream   to 100 parts
    Send 60 g

7.5 (a) Calamine   70 parts
        Arachis oil   300 parts
        Emulsifying wax   60 parts
        Water   to 1000 parts
        Send 120 g

(b) Chlorhexidine gluconate 20% solution 5 parts
    Cetomacrogol emulsifying wax   25 parts
    Liquid paraffin   10 parts
    Water   to 100 parts
    Send 30 g

(c) Zinc oxide   6 parts
    Arachis oil   7 parts
    Wool fat   2 parts
    Water   to 20 parts
    Send 60 g

(d) Calamine   7 parts
    Arachis oil   30 parts
    Emulsifying wax   6 parts
    Water   to 100 parts
    Send 150 g

(e) Chlorhexidine gluconate 20% solution 1 part
    Cetomacrogol emulsifying wax   5 parts
    Liquid paraffin   2 parts
    Water   to 20 parts
    Send 60 g

(f) Ichthammol   5 parts
    Cetostearyl alcohol   3 parts
    Wool fat   10 parts
    Zinc cream   to 100 parts
    Send 120 g

7.6 **(a)** Wool alcohols   6%
     Soft paraffin   10%
     Hard paraffin   24%
     Liquid paraffin   60%
     Send 30 g

     (b) Wool alcohols   6%
     Soft paraffin   10%
     Hard paraffin   24%
     Liquid paraffin   60%
     Send 75 g

7.7 **(a)** Menthol   2%
     Eucalyptus oil   10%
     Light magnesium carbonate   7%
     Water   to 100%
     Send 150 mL

     (b) Cetrimide   0.2%
     Cetostearyl alcohol   5%
     Liquid paraffin   50%
     Water   to 100%
     Send 120 g

     (c) Cetrimide   0.2%
     Cetostearyl alcohol   5%
     Liquid paraffin   50%
     Water   to 100%
     Send 45 g

7.8 Calculate the exact quantity of each ingredient.
     (a) Cetrimide   3%
     Cetostearyl alcohol   13.5 g
     White soft paraffin   25 g
     Liquid paraffin   to 50 g
     Send 150 g

     (b) Hydrocortisone   1%
     Clioquinol   1.5 g
     Wool fat   5 g
     White soft paraffin   to 50 g
     Send 250 g

(c) Cetomacrogol emulsifying wax   60 g
    Benzyl alcohol   3 g
    Methyl paraben   2.3%
    Water   to 200 g
    Send 40 g

(d) Cetrimide   3%
    Cetostearyl alcohol   13.5 g
    White soft paraffin   25 g
    Liquid paraffin   to 50 g
    Send 30 g

(e) Oxytetracycline   3%
    Zinc oxide   10 g
    Salicylic acid   2.5 g
    Starch   to 50 g
    Send 60 g

(f) Cetrimide   3%
    Cetostearyl alcohol   13.5 g
    White soft paraffin   25 g
    Liquid paraffin   to 50 g
    Send 40 g

(g) Cetomacrogol emulsifying wax   60 g
    Benzyl alcohol   3 g
    Methyl paraben   2.3%
    Water   to 200 g
    Send 150 g

7.9 (a) Hydrogen peroxide 20 vol   20
    Water   80
    Prepare 15 mL of eardrops

(b) Calculate the quantities to prepare 50 mL of 25 volume hydrogen peroxide from 100 volume hydrogen peroxide

7.10 This formula requires the addition of light magnesium carbonate:

    Menthol   2%
    Eucalyptus oil   10%

Water   to 100%
Send 60 mL

7.11 The following formulae require the addition of a
suspending agent:

(a) Aspirin   35 g
Chloroform water   to 1000 mL
Send 80 mL

(b) Aspirin   4%
Raspberry syrup   2.5 mL
Amaranth solution   0.1 mL
Chloroform water   to 10 mL
Send 60 mL

(c) Chalk   3 g
Syrup   20%
Cinnamon water   25%
Chloroform water   to 100 mL
Send 180 mL

(d) Aromatic chalk   9%
Opium tincture   40 mL
Catechu tincture   40 mL
Chloroform water   to 1000 mL
Send 50 mL

(e) Sulfadimidine   1.5 g
Raspberry syrup   0.4 mL
Benzoic acid solution   0.2%
Amaranth solution   0.1%
Chloroform water   to 10 mL
Send 75 mL

7.12 The following formulae require the addition of an
emulsifying agent. Also calculate the quantities for the primary
emulsions.

(a) Arachis oil   400 mL
Chloroform water   to 1000 mL
Send 100 mL
Arachis oil is a fixed oil

(b) Cod liver oil   5 mL
     Chloroform water   to 10 mL
     Send 70 mL
     Cod liver oil is a fixed oil

(c) Terebene   20 mL
     Water   to 100 mL
     Send 250 mL
     Terebene is a volatile oil

(d) Cinnamon oil   300 mL
     Water   to 1 L
     Prepare 150 mL
     Cinnamon oil is a volatile oil

(e) Halibut liver oil   50%
     Chloroform water   to 100 mL
     Send 60 mL
     Halibut liver oil is a fixed oil

(f) Liquid paraffin   50%
     Chloroform water   to 100%
     Send 50 mL
     Liquid paraffin is a mineral oil

(g) Olive oil   30%
     Water   to 10 mL
     Send 120 mL
     Olive oil is a fixed oil

(h) Calciferol   30 mL
     Chloroform water   to 1000 mL
     Send 50 mL
     Calciferol is a fixed oil

(i) Peppermint oil   1 mL
     Chloroform water   to 10 mL
     Prepare 500 mL
     Peppermint oil is a volatile oil

7.13 **(a)** Starch   7 parts
        Zinc oxide   8 parts
        Olive oil   2 parts

	Wool fat	3 parts
	Send 30 g	
(b)	Magnesium trisilicate	500 mg
	Light magnesium carbonate	750 mg
	Sodium bicarbonate	250 mg
	Chloroform water, double strength	5 mL
	Water	to 10 mL
	Send 75 mL	
(c)	Starch	350 g
	Zinc oxide	300 g
	Olive oil	200 g
	Wool fat	150 g
	Send 120 g	
(d)	Clioquinol	3%
	Cetomacrogol emulsifying wax	30%
	Chlorocresol	0.1%
	Water	to 100%
	Send 75 g	
(e)	Belladonna tincture	40 mL
	Benzoic acid solution	20 mL
	Glycerol	100 mL
	Syrup	200 mL
	Water	to 1000 mL
	Send 120 mL	
(f)	White beeswax	2 g
	Hard paraffin	3 g
	Cetostearyl alcohol	5 g
	Soft paraffin	90 g
	Send 60 g	
(g)	Light magnesium carbonate	30 g
	Sodium bicarbonate	50 g
	Aromatic cardamom tincture	30 mL
	Chloroform water, double strength	500 mL
	Water	to 1000 mL
	Send 50 mL	
(h)	Wool fat	50 parts
	Hard paraffin	25 parts

Cetostearyl alcohol 75 parts
Soft paraffin 850 parts
Send 30 g

(i) Wool alcohols 6%
Soft paraffin 10%
Hard paraffin 24%
Liquid paraffin 60%
Send 120 g

(j) Calamine 7 parts
Arachis oil 30 parts
Emulsifying wax 6 parts
Water to 100 parts
Send 240 g

(k) Cetrimide 3%
Cetostearyl alcohol 13.5 g
White soft paraffin 25 g
Liquid paraffin to 50 g
Send 120 g

(l) Magnesium sulphate 40 g
Light magnesium carbonate 5 g
Concentrated peppermint water 2.5 g
Chloroform water, double strength 30 mL
Water to 100 mL
Send 60 mL

(m) Ichthammol 25 parts
Cetostearyl alcohol 15 parts
Wool fat 50 parts
Zinc cream to 500 parts
Send 30 g

(n) Zinc oxide 30 parts
Arachis oil 35 parts
Wool fat 10 parts
Water to 100 parts
Send 150 g

(o) Hydrocortisone 1%
Clioquinol 1.5 g
Wool fat 5 g

White soft paraffin   to 50 g
Send 120 g

For answers to these questions see page 266

8 Changing concentration

After studying this chapter you will be able to:

- Use the dilution equation
- Apply the dilution equation to a range of different problems involving solid, liquid and semi-solid medicines
- Prepare flavouring waters
- Use the alligation method for dilutions and when mixing different concentrations
- Calculate dilutions involving two stages

INTRODUCTION

It is frequently necessary to change the concentration of a medicine, or an ingredient in a medicine. These changes may be to increase by the addition of more drug or, more commonly, decrease the concentration by adding a diluent. On other occasions, instructions have to be provided to the user, patient or other health professional on how to prepare the dilution for use. The types of dilution found in the reconstitution of dried medicines and their use as intravenous additives is not dealt with in this chapter, but are dealt with in Chapters 13 and 14 respectively.

It should also be remembered that, whilst dilution is most commonly encountered in liquid systems, it could also occur in solid and semi-solid systems. For example, the use of trituration, discussed in Chapter 9, is an example of preparing a dilution of a solid drug to give a diluted product from which the requisite amount of drug can be obtained. The same principles are used in the calculations for liquid, solid and semi-solid systems.

Another situation, which arises from time to time, is the need to mix two materials of different strengths to produce an intermediate strength. Older pharmacists will fondly(!) remember calculating for mixtures of different strengths of alcohol. More often it is required when commercial products are available in two strengths and the prescriber requires an intermediate strength.

In this chapter all these types of calculation will be dealt with, illustrating most of the different ways in which they may be presented. The variation arises because of the alternative ways in which the strength, of the starting system or required system, can be expressed (see Ch. 3). It is essential to ensure that units are standardized prior to starting the calculation and also to understand exactly what the problem (question) requires.

DILUTION EQUATION

Most of the problems can be solved using the dilution equation:

$$C_1 V_1 = C_2 V_2$$

where C_1 and V_1 are the initial concentration and initial volume respectively; and C_2 and V_2 are the final concentration and final volume of the mixture respectively.

When solids are being used, it is necessary to modify the equation to use weights rather than volumes:

$$C_1 W_1 = C_2 W_2$$

where W is the weight of the material.

The way of solving these problems is, therefore, to identify the values of three terms. The fourth term can be made the subject of the formula, and solved.

Example 8.1

Calculate the volume of a 5% potassium permanganate solution required to prepare 125 mL of a 0.2% solution of potassium permanganate.

Identify the terms in the dilution equation:

$$C_1 = 5\%, \ V_1 = y, \ C_2 = 0.2\%, \ V_2 = 125 \text{ mL}$$

The units of concentration are the same, and the answer will be in millilitres. These values can be substituted in the dilution equation:

$$5 \times y = 0.2 \times 125, \text{ therefore } y = \frac{0.2 \times 125}{5} = 5 \text{ mL}$$

Example 8.2

What concentration of solution is required when 10 mL diluted to 60 mL produces a 0.5% w/v solution?

Identify the values for the dilution equation:

$$C_1 = y, V_1 = 10 \text{ mL}, C_2 = 0.5\%, V_2 = 60 \text{ mL}$$

Both volumes are in millilitres, so the answer will be a percentage (weight in volume). Substituting in the dilution equation:

$$y \times 10 = 0.5 \times 60, \text{ therefore } y = \frac{0.5 \times 60}{10} = 3\% \text{ w/v}$$

Example 8.3

What volume of a 1% w/v solution is produced when 75 mL of a 5% w/v solution is diluted?

$$C_1 = 5\%, V_1 = 75 \text{ mL}, C_2 = 1.0\%, V_2 = y$$

Both concentrations are percentages, and the answer will be in millilitres:

$$5 \times 75 = 1 \times y, \text{ therefore } y = \frac{5 \times 75}{1} = 375 \text{ mL}$$

Example 8.4

What is the final concentration if 120 mL of a 12% w/v chlorhexidine solution is diluted to 240 mL with water?

$$C_1 = 12\%, V_1 = 120 \text{ mL}, C_2 = y, V_2 = 240 \text{ mL}$$

Both volumes are in millilitres and the answer will be a percentage (weight in volume):

$$12 \times 120 = y \times 240, \text{ therefore } y = \frac{12 \times 120}{240} = 6\% \text{ w/v}$$

These four examples have shown the basic, uncomplicated, calculation where the concentration in particular is expressed as a percentage. This is not always the case. It is recommended that concentrations expressed as ratio strengths be converted to percentages. Likewise, any differences in units of volume should be standardized, usually to millilitres. The following examples illustrate these processes.

Example 8.5

What concentration is produced when 200 mL of a 1 in 40 solution is diluted to 750 mL (answer to 2 decimal places)?

Convert 1 in 40 to a percentage (see Chapter 3):

$$\frac{1 \text{ part}}{40 \text{ parts}} = \frac{z \text{ parts}}{100 \text{ parts}} \text{, therefore } z = \frac{1 \times 100}{40} = 2.5 \text{ \%}$$

The dilution equation can then be applied as previously:

$$C_1 = 2.5\%, \ V_1 = 200 \text{ mL}, \ C_2 = y, \ V_2 = 750 \text{ mL}.$$

Substituting:

$$2.5 \times 200 = y \ \times 750 \text{, therefore } y = \frac{2.5 \times 200}{750} = 0.67\%$$

Note that, because the original question did not give sufficient information, it is not possible to say whether the percentage is weight in volume or volume in volume.

Example 8.6

What concentration is produced when 200 mL of a 2.5% w/v solution is diluted to 2.5 L?

Here there are two different units for volume. Convert the litres to millilitres:

$$2.5 \text{ L} = 2500 \text{ mL}$$

$$C_1 = 2.5\%, \ V_1 = 200 \text{ mL}, \ C_2 = y, \ V_2 = 2500 \text{ mL}$$

The units now correspond, with the answer being a percentage w/v. Substituting:

$$2.5 \times 200 = y \ \times 2500 \text{, therefore } y = \frac{2.5 \times 200}{2500} = 0.2\% \text{ w/v}$$

Example 8.7

Calculate the volume of a 1 in 20 solution of chlorhexidine solution required to prepare 400 mL of a 0.25% solution.

Convert 1 in 20 to percentage:

$$\frac{1 \text{ part}}{20 \text{ parts}} = \frac{z \text{ parts}}{100 \text{ parts}} \text{, therefore } z = \frac{1 \times 100}{20} = 5 \text{ \%}$$

$$C_1 = 5\%, \ V_1 = y, \ C_2 = 0.25\%, \ V_2 = 400 \text{ mL}$$

Because the units are matched, the volume will be in millilitres. Substituting in the dilution equation:

$$5 \times y = 0.25 \times 400 \text{, therefore } y = \frac{0.25 \times 400}{5} = 20 \text{ mL}$$

Example 8.8

What volume of a 0.25% solution can be prepared from 150 mL of a 1 in 80 solution?

The first step is to recognize that the missing figure from the dilution equation is the final volume (C_2). In other words, this is just another way of asking the same question which was illustrated in Example 8.3. The second step is to convert the concentration into a percentage:

$$\frac{1 \text{ part}}{80 \text{ parts}} = \frac{z \text{ parts}}{100 \text{ parts}}, \text{ therefore } z = \frac{1 \times 100}{80} = 1.25 \text{ \%}$$

$$C_1 = 1.25\%, V_1 = 150 \text{ mL}, C_2 = 0.25\%, V_2 = y$$

The answer will be in millilitres.

$$1.25 \times 150 = 0.25 \times y, \text{ therefore } y = \frac{1.25 \times 150}{0.25} = 750 \text{ mL}$$

Example 8.9

A prescription is received for 100 mL of a suspension containing 10 mg/5 mL. A commercial suspension contains 50 mg/5 mL dose. How much of the commercial suspension is required?

The concentrations here are given in weight per 5 mL dose. These could be converted into percentages, but it is easier to leave them in their present form since they both have the same units. Therefore the terms in the dilution equation can be identified.

$$C_1 = 50 \text{ mg/5 mL}, V_1 = y, C_2 = 10 \text{ mg/5 mL}, V_2 = 100 \text{ mL}$$

Substituting in the dilution equation:

$$50 \times y = 10 \times 100, \text{ therefore } y = \frac{10 \times 100}{50} = 20 \text{ mL}$$

Example 8.10

A patient is to receive a 5 mL dose containing 100 mg of drug. A 1 in 20 solution is available. How may 60 mL of the medicine be prepared?

First it is seen that we have two different ways of expressing the concentration. These must be made the same. The patient is to receive a dose of 100 mg/5 mL. This is 20 mg/1 mL, that is 2 g/100 mL—a 2% concentration. So $C_2 = 2\%$.

The 1 in 20 concentration has also to be converted to a percentage:

$$\frac{1 \text{ part}}{20 \text{ parts}} = \frac{y}{100 \text{ parts}}, \text{ therefore } y = \frac{1 \times 100}{20} = 5 \text{ \%}$$

Therefore $C_1 = 5\%$, $C_2 = 2\%$ and $V_2 = 60$ mL. Let $V_1 = y$

All the information is now ready for using the dilution equation:

$$5 \times y = 2 \times 60, \text{ therefore } y = \frac{2 \times 60}{5} = 24 \text{ mL}$$

Dilute the 1 in 20 solution with water to make 60 mL solution, and every 5 mL will contain 100 mg of drug.

Example 8.11

What percentage of atropine is produced when 150 mg of atropine powder is made up to 50 g with lactose as a diluent?

The atropine powder is a pure drug, so its concentration (C_1) is 100% w/w. The initial weight of the atropine powder (W_1) = 150 mg = 0.15 g and W_2 = 50 g. Let $C_2 = y$. Substituting in the modified dilution equation:

$$100\% \times 0.15 \text{ g} = y \times 50 \text{ g, therefore } y = \frac{100 \times 0.15}{50} = 0.3\% \text{ w/w}$$

Example 8.12

A powder mixture contains 1.0% of drug in an inert diluent. How much more diluent must be added to produce 1 kg of 1 in 2500 dispersion?

The ratio concentration must be converted to a percentage, which will be weight in weight.

$$\frac{1 \text{ part}}{2500 \text{ parts}} = \frac{z \text{ parts}}{100 \text{ parts}} \text{ , therefore } z = \frac{1 \times 100}{2500} = 0.04\% \text{ w/w}$$

We can now identify the quantities in the modified dilution equation:

$$C_1 = 1.0\%, \ W_1 = y, \ C_2 = 0.04\%, \ W_2 = 1 \text{ kg}$$

Note that the weight is in kilograms, so the answer produced will also be in kilograms. The weight could have been converted into grams if desired, but this is not necessary in this case and increases the possibility of error. Substituting:

$$1 \times y = 0.04 \times 1, \text{ therefore } y = \frac{0.04 \times 1}{1} = 0.04 \text{ kg} = 40 \text{ g}$$

Therefore, 40 g of the 1% dispersion is required which would be diluted. The amount of diluent required (call it w) can then be calculated:

$$w = (1000 - 40) = 960 \text{ g}$$

Example 8.13

An ointment is available which contains 3.5% w/w of salicylic acid in emulsifying ointment. A prescription is received for 50 g of an ointment containing 2.0% w/w salicylic acid in emulsifying ointment. How much of the 3.5% ointment and how much emulsifying ointment is required to fill this prescription?

Identify the quantities to be substituted in the modified dilution equation:

$$C_1 = 3.5\%, W_1 = y, C_2 = 2.0\%, W_2 = 50 \text{ g}$$

Substituting in the modified dilution equation:

$$3.5 \times y = 2.0 \times 50, \text{ therefore } y = \frac{2.0 \times 50}{3.5} = 28.57 \text{ g}$$

(Note: to divide by 3.5 without a calculator, it is easier to multiply top and bottom by 2, which means that the divisor will be 7.)
This is the amount of 3.5% salicylic acid ointment.
The amount of emulsifying ointment required = (50 − 28.57) = 21.43 g.
Therefore we require 28.57 g of salicylic acid ointment (3.5%) and 21.43 g of emulsifying ointment to make the prescribed ointment.

Example 8.14

Provide directions for the patient to enable them to dilute 5% potassium permanganate solution to produce 250 mL of a 0.1% solution.

The first part of the question requires the calculation of the amount of 'stock' solution required to make the dilution. This is carried out using the dilution equation:

$$C_1 = 5\%, V_1 = y \text{ mL}, C_2 = 0.1\%, V_2 = 250 \text{ mL}$$

Substituting:

$$5 \times y = 0.1 \times 250, \text{ therefore } y = \frac{0.1 \times 250}{5} = 5 \text{ mL}$$

The patient requires to dilute 5 mL to 250 mL. Assuming that the patient has a household measure they can use to measure 250 mL, the instructions will be to 'Dilute one 5 mL spoonful of the solution to 250 mL with water'.

Concentrated waters

A range of flavours is used in extemporaneously prepared medicines. These are from natural sources and are available in the form of concentrated solutions to reduce the bulk and weight during storage. These alcoholic solutions then require dilution for use using a ratio of 1 part of concentrated water plus 39 parts of water (1 part in 40).

Example 8.15

℞

Light magnesium carbonate	50 g
Sodium bicarbonate	75 g
Peppermint water	500 mL
Chloroform water	to 1000 mL

Send 200 mL

In 200 mL of suspension there is 100 mL of peppermint water. Peppermint water is only available as concentrated peppermint water. The dilution factor 1 + 39 is used.

1 mL concentrate + 39 mL water = 40 mL peppermint water

If 40 mL of peppermint water contains 1 mL of concentrated peppermint water, then 100 mL of peppermint water will contain 2.5 mL of concentrated peppermint water. Therefore to 2.5 mL of concentrated peppermint water is added 97.5 mL of water to produce the 100 mL of peppermint water required.

Example 8.16

Chloroform water is probably the most common ingredient in extemporaneously prepared mixtures, used as a flavour and preservative. As with other flavours, it is available as a concentrated solution. However, it is frequently included in master formulae as 'double strength' chloroform water. Double strength chloroform water is prepared from concentrated chloroform water by diluting in the ratio of 1 part of concentrated water to 19 parts of water (1 part in 20). The following example was used in chapter 7.

℞

Chalk	120 mg
Syrup	0.5 mL
Concentrated cinnamon water	0.02 mL
Double strength chloroform water	2.5 mL
Water	to 5 mL

Send 150 mL

This prescription requires 2.5 mL of double strength chloroform water per 5 mL, that is 75 mL in the 150 mL finished product.
The dilution of concentrated chloroform water is 1 part plus 19 parts of water, giving a total of 20 parts. To produce 75 mL, 75/20 = 3.75 mL of concentrated chloroform water would be required. Depending on the equipment available, this may be difficult to measure. In situations such as this, it is normal practice to make a small excess. In this case, making 80 mL would require 80/20 = 4 mL of concentrated chloroform water, which could be easily measured using a pipette.

ALLIGATION

Alligation is a method for solving the number of parts of two or more components of known concentration to be mixed when the final desired concentration is known. The two components may be different strengths of the same medicine, or one of them can be the pure drug—which has a concentration of 100%.

To use, the information is laid out in the following way:

Starting concentration (A)   Difference between (B) and (C)

Target concentration (C)

Starting concentration (B)   Difference between (A) and (C)

The numerical difference between (B) and (C) indicates the number of parts of (A) which is required, whilst the numerical difference between (A) and (C) indicates the number of parts of (B) which is required. The mathematical basis for the alligation method can be found in books such as *Cooper and Gunn's Dispensing for Pharmaceutical Students* (Gunn & Carter 1965). The following example demonstrates its use in practice.

Example 8.17

Calculate the amount of salicylic acid that must be added to 50 g of a 1.5% w/w ointment to produce a 4% w/w ointment.

Salicylic acid is entered as 100%.

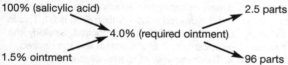

100% (salicylic acid)   2.5 parts

4.0% (required ointment)

1.5% ointment   96 parts

As shown above, the difference between the concentration of the pure drug powder (100%, recorded top left) and the desired concentration (4%) is 96 (recorded bottom right). This is equivalent to the number of parts of 1.5% ointment required (read horizontally across the bottom). Similarly, the difference between the concentration of 1.5% ointment (recorded bottom left) and the desired concentration (4%) is 2.5 (recorded top right). This is equivalent to the number of parts of 100% drug (salicylic acid) needed for the mixture (read horizontally across the top).

Therefore we require 2.5 parts of salicylic acid and 96 parts of 1.5% w/w ointment.

The question indicates that there are 50 g of the 1.5% ointment. Therefore 50 g = 96 parts.

Using simple proportion, letting the amount of salicylic acid required be y, we have:

$$\frac{50}{96} = \frac{y}{2.5}, \text{ therefore } y = \frac{50 \times 2.5}{96} = 1.30 \text{ g (to 2 decimal places)}$$

Therefore we require 1.30 g salicylic acid added to 50 g of 1.5% w/w salicylic acid ointment to produce the requested 4.0% w/w salicylic acid ointment.

Note: As with many calculations, it is possible to check that the answer is correct by 'working backwards'. 50 g of 1.5% ointment contains 0.75 g of salicylic acid. We are going to add 1.30 g, to give a total of 2.05 g of salicylic acid. This is contained in the new total weight of 51.3 g of ointment (50 + 1.30). When we calculate the percentage we find that it is 4.00% (to 2 decimal places), confirming that the answer is correct.

Example 8.18

Calculate the amounts of 2% w/w metronidazole cream and metronidazole powder required to produce 150 g of 6% w/w metronidazole cream (to 2 decimal places).

This question is slightly different in that a specific amount of finished ointment is specified. This requires a slightly different handling of the 'parts' once they have been obtained by alligation as follows:

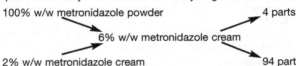

100% w/w metronidazole powder   4 parts

6% w/w metronidazole cream

2% w/w metronidazole cream   94 parts

As shown above, the difference between the concentration of the pure drug powder (100%) and the desired concentration (6%) is 94. This is equivalent to the number of parts of 2% cream required. Similarly, the difference between the concentration of 2% cream and the desired concentration (6%) is 4. This is equivalent to the number of parts of 100% drug (metronidazole powder) needed for the mixture.

The total amount (4 parts + 94 parts = 98 parts) is 150 g.

Thus, 1 part = 150/98 g.

Therefore, the amount of 2% cream
required = 94 parts × 150/98 g = 143.88 g.

The amount of pure metronidazole (100%)
required = 4 parts × 150/98 g = 6.12 g.

Note: The accuracy of the answer can be checked. 143.88 g of 2% cream contain 2.88 g of metronidazole (to 2 decimal places), to which we are adding 6.12 g, giving a total of 9.00 g of metronidazole. This is in 150 g, which is 6% w/w as requested.

Example 8.19

Thioridazine suspension is available as Melleril® Suspension at concentrations of 25 mg/5 mL and 100 mg/5 mL. Calculate the quantities to use to prepare 100 mL of 40 mg/5 mL suspension.

It is not necessary to convert the concentrations to percentages. Use the numbers of milligrams in 5 mL as the figures for the subtractions. Using the alligation method:

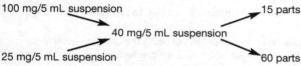

Total number of parts = 15 parts + 60 parts = 75 parts, which is equivalent to 100 mL. Using simple proportion we can calculate:

$$\text{Amount of 100 mg/5 mL thioridazine suspension} = \frac{15 \times 100}{75} = 20 \text{ mL}$$

$$\text{Amount of 25 mg/5 mL thioridazine suspension} = \frac{60 \times 100}{75} = 80 \text{ mL}$$

Example 8.20

The dispensary has stocks of 3% w/w sulphur ointment and 8% w/w sulphur ointment. A prescription arrives for 30 g of 6.5% sulphur ointment. Calculate the quantities to be used.

There are several possible ways in which this could be calculated. If sulphur is available, it could be added to the 3% w/w sulphur ointment, using the method shown in Example 8.18. If the vehicle for the ointment is available, the 8% w/w sulphur ointment could be diluted. The third method is to mix the two available ointments in an appropriate proportion to be determined using alligation:

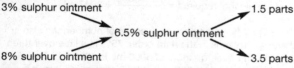

From the right-hand side we see that there are 5 parts (1.5 + 3.5), which are equivalent to the 30 g ointment required. We can use simple proportion to calculate the actual quantities:

$$\text{1.5 parts of 3% sulphur ointment} = \frac{1.5 \times 30}{5} = 9.0 \text{ g}$$

$$2.5 \text{ parts of 8\% sulphur ointment} = \frac{3.5 \times 30}{5} = 21.0 \text{ g}$$

We can observe that the total weight of the two ointments being used adds up to 30 g. We can also calculate the weight of sulphur in 9 g of 3% ointment (0.27 g) and in 21 g of 8% ointment (1.68 g), that is a total of 1.95 g of sulphur will be in the finished ointment. 30 g of 6.5% sulphur ointment is required to contain 1.95 g, confirming the accuracy of the calculation.

Example 8.21

What volume of 95% alcohol is required to produce 5 L of 75% alcohol?

This calculation can be carried out using the dilution equation or using alligation (taking water as 0% ingredient).

(a) Dilution equation

Identify the terms in the dilution equation:

$$C_1 = 95\%, V_1 = y, C_2 = 75\%, V_2 = 5000 \text{ mL}$$

Substituting:

$$95 \times y = 75 \times 5000, \text{ therefore } y, = \frac{75 \times 5000}{95} = 3947 \text{ mL}$$

(b) Alligation

Set out the alligation calculation:

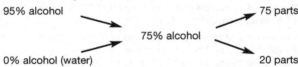

95% alcohol   75 parts

75% alcohol

0% alcohol (water)   20 parts

There are a total of 95 parts, which are equivalent to 5000 mL, therefore we can calculate the amount of 95% alcohol:

$$95\% \text{ alcohol required} = \frac{75 \times 5000}{95} = 3947 \text{ mL}$$

Both methods give the same answer. A sense of number can also indicate that the answer is in the right order. 75% is a little over three quarters of 95% and three quarters of 5000 mL is 3750 mL. The answer, therefore should be a little over this figure, which it is. It is also possible to calculate the amount of alcohol and confirm the answer that way.

Example 8.22

What volumes of 95% alcohol and 43% alcohol are required to produce 5 L of 75% alcohol?

Because we do not have a pure diluent as the second ingredient, we cannot now use the dilution equation. However, the alligation method works:

95% alcohol ⟶ 32 parts

75% alcohol

43% alcohol ⟶ 20 parts

There are 52 parts, which are equivalent to 5000 mL:

Amount of 95% alcohol $= \dfrac{32 \times 5000}{52} = 3077$ mL (rounded to 4 significant figures)

Amount of 43% alcohol $= \dfrac{20 \times 5000}{52} = 1923$ mL (rounded to 4 significant figures)

It can be seen that the volumes add up to 5000 mL. Calculation of the amount of alcohol would confirm the accuracy of the calculation.

COMPLEX DILUTION

Sometimes questions are asked where the use of the dilution equation is not easily applied. These are illustrated in the remaining examples of this chapter. The important aspect to answering them correctly is to identify exactly what the question is asking. Until you are confident, it is also possible to calculate 'backwards' to confirm that the correct answer has been achieved.

Example 8.23

What volume of a 2% w/v solution is required to prepare 200 mL of a solution such that a 1 in 20 dilution will produce a 1 in 5000 solution? The first step is to convert the ratio concentration into a percentage:

$$\frac{1}{5000} = \frac{z}{100} \text{, therefore } z = \frac{100 \times 1}{5000} = 0.02\%$$

The next stage is to attempt to identify the terms in the dilution equation:
$C_1 = 2\%$ w/v, $V_1 =$ is unknown, call it y, C_2 is not clear: the question indicates a 1 in 20 dilution produces a 0.02% solution, $V_2 = 200$ mL. The main problem is in clarifying the value of C_2. The concentration required is 20 times more concentrated than the final 0.02%. This is

because, after the 20 fold dilution, a 0.02% solution must result. Therefore the value for C_2 will be $0.02 \times 20 = 0.4\%$ w/v. The dilution equation can now be used:

$$2 \times y = 0.4 \times 200, \text{ therefore } y = \frac{0.4 \times 200}{2} = 40 \text{ mL}$$

By working backwards the answer can be checked by calculating how much drug is in 200 mL of 0.4% solution:

$$\text{Amount of drug} = \frac{200 \times 0.4}{100} = 0.8 \text{ g}$$

40 mL of 2% solution contains 0.8 g.

There are different ways of carrying out this type of calculation. The following example will be used to show another approach.

Example 8.24

What weight of potassium permanganate is required to produce 500 mL of a solution so that when 5 mL of solution is diluted to 200 mL with water it produces a 0.05% w/v solution?

Calculate the amount of potassium permanganate in 200 mL of 0.05% solution. Let the amount of potassium permanganate = y, therefore:

$$\frac{y}{200} = \frac{0.05}{100} \text{ , therefore } y = \frac{0.05 \times 200}{100} = 0.1 \text{ g}$$

This 0.1 g is contained in the 5 mL which is taken from the concentrated solution. Therefore, the concentrated solution contains 0.1 g in 5 mL. This can be converted to a percentage ($0.1 \times 20 = 2\%$), and the weight required for 500 mL of this solution calculated:

$$= \frac{2 \times 500}{100} = 10 \text{ g}$$

or it can be seen that, since 500 mL is required, we required:

$$= \frac{500 \times 0.1}{5} = 10 \text{ g}.$$

Therefore, 10 g of potassium permanganate are dissolved in 500 mL to form the concentrated solution; 5 mL of this concentrate, diluted to 200 mL, produces a 0.05% w/v solution.

Example 8.25

Prepare 80 mL of 1% w/v potassium permanganate solution. Give instructions to the patient to produce 1 L of 0.1 mg/1 mL of potassium permanganate solution.

First, work out the quantity of potassium permanganate required to make the concentrated solution.

Let the quantity of potassium permanganate required = y. Thus:

$$\frac{y}{80} = \frac{1}{100} \text{ , therefore } y = \frac{1 \times 80}{100} = 0.8 \text{ g}$$

Second, convert the concentration of the dilute solution into a percentage.

To convert the quantities into 100 mL, multiply by 100, therefore 100×0.1 mg = 10 mg/100 mL.

Divide by 1000 to convert to grams:

$$\frac{10 \text{ mg/100 mL}}{1000} = 0.01 \text{ g/100 mL}$$

Therefore, the dilute solution is 0.01% w/v.

The dilution process involves moving from a 1% w/v solution to a 0.01% solution. This is a 1 in 100 dilution. In other words, the volume of concentrated solution required will be one hundredth of the final volume of diluted solution. Therefore:

$$\text{Volume of concentrated solution} = \frac{1000}{100} = 10 \text{ mL}$$

The answers to the two parts of the question are:

Dissolve 0.8 g potassium permanganate in water and make up to 80 mL with water. The instructions to the patient are to 'Dilute two 5 mL spoonfuls to 1 litre with water for use'. As with previous calculations, this can be worked backwards to confirm the answer. 1 L of 0.1 mg/1 mL solution contains 0.1×1000 mg of potassium permanganate = 100 mg. This quantity should be in the 10 mL used for dilution.

$$10 \text{ mL of 1\% solution contains } \frac{10}{100} = 0.1 \text{ g of potassium}$$

$$\text{permanganate} = 100 \text{ mg}$$

It follows that the required amount of potassium permanganate is contained in 10 mL of the concentrated solution.

SELF-STUDY QUESTIONS

8.1 What concentration is produced by the following dilutions? (To 2 decimal places)

(a) 60 mL of a 10% solution diluted to 750 mL

(b) 200 mL of a 2.5% solution diluted to 2000 mL

(c) 100 mL of a 5% solution diluted to 750 mL

(d) 150 mL of a 2.5% solution diluted to 2 L

(e) 150 mL of a 4% solution diluted to 1500 mL

(f) 75 mL of an 8% solution diluted to 500 mL

8.2 What is the final concentration of the following dilutions?

(a) 60 mL of a 1 in 10 solution diluted to 750 mL

(b) 150 mL of a 1 in 25 solution diluted to 500 mL

(c) 75 mL of a 1 in 12.5 solution diluted to 1250 mL

(d) 150 mL of a 1 in 25 solution diluted to 3 L

(e) 60 mL of a 1 in 10 solution diluted to 1.5 L

(f) 200 mL of a 1 in 40 solution diluted to 1250 mL

8.3 What volume of each solution can be produced by the following dilutions?

(a) 0.25% from 150 mL of 1 in 20 solution

(b) 1% from 225 mL of 1 in 30 solution

(c) 0.5% from 300 mL of 1 in 40 solution

(d) 1.5% from 300 mL of 1 in 25 solution

(e) 0.8% from 300 mL of 1 in 60 solution

8.4 What volume of each solution can be made by the following dilutions?

(a) 1.5% from 75 mL of 5% solution

(b) 2% from 75 mL of 5% solution

(c) 3% from 75 mL of 5% solution

(d) 3% from 150 mL of 5% solution

(e) 3.75% from 150 mL of 5% solution

(f) 2% from 225 mL of 5% solution

(g) 1.5% from 300 mL of 2.5% solution

8.5 Calculate the final concentration of the following dilutions:

(a) 150 mL of a 2.5% solution is diluted to 1000 mL

(b) 150 mL of a 4% solution is diluted to 500 mL

(c) 125 mL of an 8% solution is diluted to 500 mL

(d) 75 mL of an 8% solution is diluted to 3 L

(e) 60 mL of a 10% solution is diluted to 1 L.

8.6   What concentration of solution is produced by the following dilutions?

(a)   150 mL of a 1 in 25 solution is diluted to 3 L
(b)   75 mL of a 1 in 12.5 solution is diluted to 500 mL
(c)   60 mL of a 1 in 10 solution is diluted to 500 mL
(d)   200 mL of a 1 in 40 solution is diluted to 1000 mL
(e)   200 mL of a 1 in 40 solution is diluted to 1250 mL

8.7   What volume of each solution can be made from the given amount of concentrated solution?

(a)   1.25% solution from 300 mL of 125 mg/5 mL solution
(b)   0.75% solution from 150 mL of 50 mg/mL solution
(c)   0.8% solution from 300 mL of 25 mg/mL solution
(d)   0.5% solution from 300 mL of 50 mg/2 mL solution
(e)   0.25% solution from 150 mL of 0.25 mg/5 mL solution
(f)   1% solution from 225 mL of 250 mg/5 mL solution
(g)   3.75% solution from 225 mL of 100 mg/2 mL solution
(h)   1.2% solution from 300 mL of 125 mg/5 mL solution
(i)   0.75% solution from 150 mL of 500 mg/10 mL solution

8.8   Calculate the volume of potassium permanganate solution required to produce each dilute solution:

(a)   5% solution to prepare 100 mL of a 0.25% solution
(b)   5% solution to prepare 125 mL of a 0.2% solution
(c)   5% solution to prepare 500 mL of a 0.1% solution
(d)   5% solution to prepare 750 mL of a 0.1% solution
(e)   5% solution to prepare 400 mL of a 0.25% solution
(f)   4% solution to prepare 200 mL of a 0.1% solution
(g)   4% solution to prepare 400 mL of a 0.2% solution
(h)   4% solution to prepare 240 mL of a 0.25% solution
(i)   4% solution to prepare 600 mL of a 0.1% solution
(j)   4% solution to prepare 120 mL of a 0.5% solution

8.9   Calculate the volume of cetrimide concentrate required to produce each dilute solution:

(a)   4% solution to prepare 200 mL of 1 in 1000 solution
(b)   4% solution to prepare 100 mL of 1 in 500 solution

(c) 4% solution to prepare 400 mL of 1 in 500 solution

(d) 4% solution to prepare 600 mL of 1 in 1000 solution

8.10 Calculate the volume of chlorhexidine concentrate required to produce each dilute solution:

(a) 1 in 20 solution to prepare 1000 mL of a 0.1% solution

(b) 1 in 20 solution to prepare 50 mL of a 0.5% solution

(c) 1 in 25 solution to prepare 200 mL of a 0.1% solution

(d) 1 in 25 solution to prepare 100 mL of a 0.2% solution

(e) 1 in 25 solution to prepare 600 mL of a 0.1% solution

(f) 1 in 20 solution to prepare 250 mL of a 0.2% solution

8.11 What percentage is produced by each dilution?

(a) 150 mg of powder made up to 50 g with a diluent

(b) 150 mg of powder made up to 75 g with a diluent

(c) 200 mg of powder made up to 40 g with a diluent

(d) 300 mg of powder made up to 120 g with a diluent

(e) 450 mg of powder made up to 25 g with a diluent

8.12 How much drug is required to prepare each mixture?

(a) 250 g of a 0.08% w/w   (d) 75 g of a 0.2% w/w

(b) 25 g of a 0.8% w/w   (e) 80 g of a 0.25% w/w

(c) 50 g of a 0.6% w/w   (f) 150 g of a 0.13% w/w

8.13 How much drug is required to prepare each mixture?

(a) 40 g of a 1 in 200   (e) 90 g of a 1 in 200

(b) 75 g of a 1 in 250   (f) 120 g of a 1 in 800

(c) 120 g of a 1 in 400   (g) 30 g of a 1 in 200

(d) 30 g of a 1 in 100

8.14 Calculate the amount of concentrated peppermint water required to make 60 mL of peppermint water.

8.15 120 mL of chloroform water is required. How much concentrated chloroform water should be diluted with water?

8.16 It is estimated that 70 mL of cinnamon water will be required for an extemporaneous preparation. Suggest how this should be prepared from concentrated cinnamon water.

8.17 How much concentrated anise water is required to make 100 mL of single strength anise water?

8.18 A formula requires 2.5 mL of double strength peppermint water in 5 mL. The prescription requires 50 mL to be dispensed. How much concentrated peppermint water is required?

8.19 Calculate the quantity of concentrated chloroform water required to prepare 1 L of double strength chloroform water.

8.20 In dispensing a mixture, 500 mL of double strength cinnamon water is required in 1 L and 150 mL is to be provided. Suggest how this might be prepared from concentrated cinnamon water.

8.21 What weight of drug must be added to produce the required strength of ointment? (To 2 decimal places):

(a) 50 g of 2% ointment to produce a 3% ointment
(b) 50 g of 2.5% ointment to produce a 4% ointment
(c) 50 g of 2% ointment to produce a 3.5% ointment
(d) 150 g of 2.5% ointment to produce a 3% ointment
(e) 150 g of 1% ointment to produce a 4% ointment
(f) 150 g of 3.5% ointment to produce a 4% ointment
(g) 100 g of 2% ointment to produce a 3.5% ointment
(h) 200 g of 2.5% ointment to produce a 3.5% ointment
(i) 150 g of 1.5% ointment to produce a 4.5% ointment

8.22 Calculate the amount of drug and initial ointment to be mixed to produce the following ointments:

(a) 2% w/w ointment to make 150 g of 3% ointment
(b) 1% w/w ointment to make 150 g of 3% ointment
(c) 1.5% w/w ointment to make 100 g of 4% ointment

(d) 1% w/w ointment to make 200 g of 3.5% ointment

(e) 2.5% w/w ointment to make 60 g of 3.5% ointment

(f) 1.5% w/w ointment to make 90 g of 4.5% ointment

(g) 1% w/w ointment to make 50 g of 3% ointment

(h) 2.5% w/w ointment to make 120 g of 3% ointment

(i) 3.5% w/w ointment to make 75 g of 4% ointment

8.23 Thioridazine syrup is available as 25 mg/5 mL and 100 mg/5 mL. Calculate the quantities to use to prepare the following prescribed medicines:

(a) 100 mL of 40 mg/5 mL syrup

(b) 200 mL of 50 mg/5 mL syrup

8.24 Sulphur ointment is available as 5% w/w and 8% w/w. Calculate the quantities to use in order to prepare the following specified ointments:

(a) 30 g of 6.5% w/w ointment

(b) 60 g of 6% w/w ointment

(c) 60 g of 7.5% w/w ointment

8.25 Orphenadrine syrup is available as 25 mg/5 mL and 50 mg/5 mL. Calculate the quantities to use to prepare the following prescribed amounts:

(a) 50 mL of 30 mg/5 mL syrup

(b) 100 mL of 35 mg/5 mL syrup

(c) 1000 mL of 45 mg/5 mL syrup

8.26 Ichthammol ointment is available as 5% w/w and 7.5% w/w. Calculate the quantities to use to prepare each of the following ointments:

(a) 30 g of 5.5% w/w ointment

(b) 60 g of 6.5% w/w ointment

(c) 120 g of 6% w/w ointment

8.27 Calculate the volumes of the two strengths of alcohol available to prepare the required volume of the new concentration of alcohol:

(a) 95% alcohol and 30% alcohol to prepare 100 mL of 80% alcohol
(b) 50% alcohol and 95% alcohol to prepare 250 mL of 59% alcohol
(c) 75% alcohol and 59% alcohol to prepare 80 mL of 68% alcohol
(d) 20% alcohol and 95% alcohol to prepare 120 mL of 40% alcohol
(e) 95% alcohol and water to prepare 2000 mL of 40% alcohol

8.28 An injection of amphotericin contains 50 mg/10 mL. What volume must be added to a normal saline infusion to provide the specified total dose?

(a) 500 mL to provide 11.5 mg dose
(b) 250 mL to provide 6 mg dose
(c) 100 mL to provide 15 mg dose
(d) 750 mL to provide 17.5 mg dose
(e) 300 mL to provide 10 mg dose
(f) 1000 mL to provide 25 mg dose

8.29 An injection of Polymyxin B sulphate contains 250 000 units/5 mL. What volume is added to normal saline to give the required infusion?

(a) 500 mL infusion containing 120 000 units
(b) 250 mL infusion containing 135 000 units
(c) 1000 mL infusion containing 165 000 units

8.30 In preparing an IV infusion, you have a sterile solution containing the drug. What volume must be added to a 500 mL infusion to provide the specified total dose (to 2 decimal places)?

(a) 1 g/mL adrenaline hydrochloride (epinephrine hydrochloride) ($C_9H_{13}NO_3$.HCl) to provide a 10 mmol total dose

(b) 2 g/mL cefuroxime axetil ($C_{20}H_{22}N_4O_{10}S$) to provide a 20 mmol total dose

(c) 4 g/mL furosemide (frusemide) ($C_{12}H_{11}ClN_2O_5S$) to provide a 15 mmol total dose

(d) 0.5 g/mL chloramphenicol ($C_{11}H_{12}Cl_2N_2O_5$) to provide a 12 mmol total dose

(e) 3 g/mL cefotaxime sodium ($C_{16}H_{16}N_5NaO_7S_2$) to provide a 15 mmol total dose

(f) 2 g/mL cortisone ($C_{21}H_{28}O_5$) to provide a 20 mmol total dose

8.31 Calculate the strength of a solution such that when the specified volume is diluted as indicated, the required concentration is produced:

(a) 5 mL when diluted to 1 L produces a 1 in 10 000 solution

(b) 15 mL when diluted to 1 L produces a 1 in 750 solution

8.32 How much potassium permanganate is required to make 50 mL of a solution which, when diluted as shown, gives the indicated final solution?

(a) 5 mL diluted to 20 mL produces a 0.5% solution

(b) 5 mL diluted to 600 mL produces a 1 in 5000 solution

8.33 How much cetrimide is required to make 30 mL of a solution which, when 1 mL is diluted to 100 mL, produces a 100 parts per million solution?

8.34 How much of a 0.5% solution is required so that when diluted to 600 mL it produces a 1 in 8000 solution?

8.35 How much of a 2.0% solution when diluted to 1 L produces a 0.01% solution?

8.36 Calculate the following:

(a) What volume of 0.8% solution can be made from 300 mL of 2.5% solution?

(b) What concentration of solution is required so that when 200 mL is diluted to 1500 mL a 1 in 40 solution is produced?

(c) An injection of amphotericin contains 50 mg/10 mL. What volume must be added to 500 mL of normal saline infusion to provide a 13.5 mg total dose?

(d) Orphenadrine syrup is available as 25 mg/5 mL and 50 mg/5 mL. Calculate the quantities to use to prepare 50 mL of 35 mg/5 mL syrup.

(e) Calculate the amount of drug and 3.5% w/w ointment required to make 150 g of 4% ointment.

(f) How much drug is required to prepare 25 g of a 1.2% w/w mixture?

(g) What quantities of 95% alcohol and 45% alcohol are required to prepare 150 mL of 72% alcohol?

(h) What weight of drug must be added to 50 g of 3% ointment to produce a 5.5% ointment?

(i) What percentage is produced when 150 mg of powder is made up to 90 g with a diluent?

(j) How much benzalkonium chloride is required to make 60 mL of a solution which, when 15 mL is diluted to 150 mL, produces a 1 in 1250 solution?

(k) What concentration is produced when 150 mL of a 2.5% solution is diluted to 900 mL?

(l) Calculate the volume of a 1 in 20 solution of chlorhexidine solution required to prepare 100 mL of a 0.5% solution.

(m) In preparing an IV infusion, you have a solution containing 2 g/mL erythromycin (molecular weight 733.9). What volume must be added to a 500 mL infusion to provide a 10 mmol total dose?

(n) How much drug is required to prepare 180 g of a 1 in 400 mixture?

(o) An injection of Polymyxin B sulphate contains 500 000 units/10 mL. What volume must be added to 500 mL of normal saline infusion to produce an infusion containing 157 500 units?

(p) What weight of drug must be added to 50 g of 1.5% ointment to produce a 4% ointment?

(q) What volume of a 2% solution can be produced from 300 mL of 250 mg/10 mL solution?

(r) How much potassium permanganate is required to make 50 mL of a 0.025% solution? Calculate how much of this solution is required so that, when diluted to 20 mL, it produces a 1 in 40 000 solution.

(s) Thioridazine syrup is available as 25 mg/5 mL and 100 mg/5 mL. Calculate the quantities to use to prepare 200 mL of 40 mg/5 mL syrup.

(t) What concentration is produced when 150 mL of a 1 in 25 solution is diluted to 1500 mL?

(u) What volume of a 1.5% solution can be produced from 225 mL of 1 in 20 solution?

(v) Calculate the volume of a 5% potassium permanganate solution required to prepare 50 mL of a 0.5% solution.

(w) What percentage is produced when 450 mg of powder is made up to 30 g with a diluent?

(x) Calculate the final concentration when 75 mL of an 8% solution is diluted to 2 L.

(y) A formula requires 50 mL of double strength chloroform water. How can this be prepared from concentrated chloroform water?

(z) Calculate the volume of 4% solution of cetrimide required to prepare 800 mL of 1 in 1000 solution.

For answers to these questions see page 277

Trituration

After studying this chapter you will be able to:

- **Calculate a trituration for a solution**
- **Calculate a trituration for a powder**
- **Calculate triturations from manufactured tablets and capsules**

Balances and measures do not have limitless accuracy or sensitivity. In the context of extemporaneous dispensing, pharmacists may be required to weigh or measure quantities which are too small to be measured accurately on the equipment available.

Liquid measuring equipment may be measures or (micro)pipettes. By selection of the appropriate device, there is not normally a problem in measuring liquids with sufficient accuracy in extemporaneous dispensing.

The traditional 'Class B' dispensing balance can only be used for weighing down to 100 mg, and in increments of 10 mg above that weight. Modern electronic balances have a wider range and greater sensitivity, but would not normally be used for quantities less than 20 mg. If a small quantity of drug is required, an excess of drug must be dissolved or mixed with a suitable diluent, from which an appropriate quantity can be taken to provide the required amount of drug. This process is called trituration.

TRITURATION FOR A SOLUTION

If the quantity of drug to be incorporated into a solution is too small to weigh, the minimum weighable quantity is weighed out (100 mg on a traditional balance) and dissolved in the solvent which is to be used for the final solution (frequently water or chloroform water). An aliquot of this solution, which contains the required amount of drug, is removed and diluted to the final volume with the solvent.

Example 9.1
Calculate the quantities required to prepare 100 mL of a solution containing 2.5 mg morphine hydrochloride per 5 mL.

Quantities for 100 mL:
Morphine hydrochloride   50 mg
Chloroform water   to 100 mL

The solubility of morphine hydrochloride is 1 in 24 of water.
The minimum quantity of 100 mg of morphine hydrochloride is weighed and made up to 10 mL with chloroform water (this weight of morphine hydrochloride will dissolve in 2.4 mL).
5 mL of this solution (A) provides the 50 mg of morphine hydrochloride required.
Take 5 mL of solution A (measured using a pipette for accuracy) and make up to 100 mL with chloroform water.
Example 9.1 is a general method which will work for most situations. However, care is required to ensure that the drug is soluble in the volume of solvent being used (see Ch. 6). If required, larger volumes of solvent can be used, although the aim should always be to minimize the waste involved, i.e. use the minimum weight of drug (100 mg) and volume of solvent.

TRITURATION FOR POWDERS

For most practical extemporaneous dispensing the minimum weighable quantity is taken to be 100 mg. Additionally, *The Pharmaceutical Codex* indicates that the final powder should not weigh less than 120 mg. In making dilutions of powders, an inert solid is needed as diluent. This is normally lactose, but other powders can be used if required or more suitable (for example in lactose intolerance). As a general rule, dilutions are made in the ratio of 1 part of drug plus 9 parts of diluent—that is 100 mg of drug plus 900 mg of diluent.

Example 9.2

℞

Digoxin   0.5 mg
Make a powder
Send 24
Label: 1 daily

When making individual powders like this, it is advisable to make a small excess to allow for losses. Here, two extra powders would be suitable, so calculate for 26 powders:

Weight of digoxin required is $0.5 \times 26 = 13$ mg

This cannot be weighed, so a trituration is made, using lactose to produce a more dilute powder.

Digoxin   100 mg
Lactose   900 mg

Thus there is 100 mg digoxin in 1000 mg of mixture. Therefore, there are 10 mg digoxin in 100 mg of mixture.
We require 13 mg of digoxin. This is contained in:

$$\frac{100 \times 13}{10} = 130 \text{ mg mixture.}$$

This quantity can be weighed on a dispensing balance. Each powder should weigh 120 mg. Therefore the total weight of powder is $26 \times 120 = 3120$ mg.
We have 130 mg of powder mixture. Therefore to make the final mixture, we require $3120 - 130$ mg = 2990 mg of lactose.
To complete the process, 2990 mg (2.99 g) of lactose is added (by doubling up) to 130 mg of the digoxin and lactose mixture. Each powder weighs 120 mg and contains 0.5 mg digoxin.

Example 9.3

Let us now suppose that the same prescription is received, but for 14 powders.

℞

Digoxin   0.5 mg
Make a powder
Send 14
Label: 1 daily

An excess of 2 powders is made (16 powders).
The weight of final powder required will be 16×120 mg = 1920 mg.
The amount of digoxin required is 16×0.5 mg = 8 mg digoxin.

Weigh   100 mg digoxin
Mix with   900 mg lactose

Therefore, 10 mg of digoxin is contained in 100 mg of mixture. To obtain 8 mg of digoxin we would require:

$$\frac{100 \times 8}{10} = 80 \text{ mg of this mixture.}$$

We cannot weigh 80 mg because it is less than 100 mg. Therefore we have to make a further dilution. Call the first mixture Mixture A.

| Weigh | 100 mg Mixture A (contains 10 mg digoxin) |
| Mix with | 900 mg lactose |

Therefore, 1 mg of digoxin is contained in 100 mg of this mixture— Mixture B. To obtain 8 mg digoxin, we require:

$$\frac{100 \times 8}{1} = 800 \text{ mg Mixture B.}$$

This quantity can be weighed and made up to a final weight (1920 mg) with lactose (1920 − 800 = 1120 mg).

Note: The quantity of drug in 100 mg of Mixture A was greater than the target weight, so a further dilution was required. However, in Mixture B the weight of drug in 100 mg was less than the target, so the required amount could be weighed. As a general rule, when the amount of drug required is contained in less than 100 mg further dilutions are required. In more general terms, continue to dilute until the amount of drug in the minimum weighable quantity is less than the target weight (see Example 9.4.)

Example 9.4

If the same prescription were received for just 1 powder, similar processes could be carried out. (Assume that no excess is being made.)

Mixture A:

| Weigh | 100 mg of digoxin |
| Mix with | 900 mg lactose |

Mixture B:

| Weigh | 100 mg Mixture A (contains 10 mg digoxin in 100 mg) |
| Mix with | 900 mg lactose |

Mixture C:

| Weigh | 100 mg Mixture B (contains 1 mg digoxin in 100 mg) |
| Mix with | 900 mg lactose |

In Mixture C 100 mg contains 0.1 mg digoxin. This is less than the target weight of 0.5 mg, therefore the trituration can be completed with this dilution.

The required digoxin is in:

$$\frac{100 \times 0.5 \text{ mg}}{0.1} = 500 \text{ mg Mixture C.}$$

An alternative conclusion to this dilution is as follows:

Weigh   100 mg Mixture B (contains 1 mg digoxin in 100 mg)
Mix with   100 mg lactose.

Now 1 mg digoxin is contained in 200 mg, therefore 0.5 mg digoxin is contained in 100 mg of powder.

The final weight should be made up to at least 120 mg. However, it should be noted that a single powder such as this would not be prepared. It was used as an example to show how a series of triturations can be made if required.

TRITURATIONS FROM MANUFACTURED MEDICINES

It can happen that the exact dose required for a child is not available in a manufactured medicine, nor is the drug available for the pharmacist to make a preparation of the required strength. In such situations, it is necessary to use manufactured tablets or capsules as the source of the drug, providing these are not modified-release preparations. Tablets would be crushed, whilst capsules would be emptied. The resulting powder then has to be weighed, because there are other ingredients present. From the amount of drug claimed on the label and the actual weight, it is possible to carry out the dilution.

Example 9.5

A child, weight 5 kg, is to receive spironolactone 3 mg/kg three times daily. Tablets containing 25 mg, 50 mg and 100 mg are available. Calculate the quantities to be used in powder to provide 20 doses.

The individual dose for the child will be 5×3 mg = 15 mg (see Chs 11 and 12). This is not directly available in a manufactured form, therefore a trituration will be made.

Total weight of spironolactone required will be $15 \times 20 = 300$ mg. This can be made from 3×100 mg tablets (or 6×50 mg). Take the tablets, weigh them—say they weigh 354 mg—then crush them to a powder. The minimum amount for the powders will be 120 mg, therefore the total weight of powder mixture should be $20 \times 120 = 2400$ mg = 2.4 g.

The weight of diluent (lactose) to be added will be (2400 – 354) = 2046 mg. Alternatively, diluent can be added to give a final weight of 2.4 g (with mixing by doubling-up during the addition).
Individual powders of 120 mg are weighed and wrapped.

SELF-STUDY QUESTIONS

Calculate for the number of powders indicated (do not make for an excess). Assume that the minimum weighable quantity is 100 mg. Answers should be given to the nearest 10 mg.

9.1 Calculate a method for preparing the following aqueous solutions:
- **(a)** 7 × 5 mL doses of atropine sulphate solution containing 1 mg/5 mL (Solubility 1 in 0.5)
- **(b)** 10 × 5 mL doses of ergotamine tartrate solution containing 2 mg/5 mL (Solubility 1 in 500)
- **(c)** 10 × 5 mL doses of morphine sulphate solution containing 2.5 mg/5 mL (Solubility 1 in 21)
- **(d)** 10 × 5 mL doses of hyoscine hydrobromide solution containing 500 µg/5 mL (Solubility 1 in 3.5)
- **(e)** 7 × 5 mL doses of morphine sulphate solution containing 2.5 mg/5 mL (Solubility 1 in 21)
- **(f)** 10 × 5 mL doses of codeine phosphate solution containing 3 mg/5 mL (Solubility 1 in 4)
- **(g)** 7 × 5 mL doses of hyoscine hydrobromide solution containing 500 µg/5 mL (Solubility 1 in 3.5).

9.2 Calculate a trituration to make each of the following prescriptions:
- **(a)** 20 × 120 mg powders, each containing 0.6 mg of hyoscine hydrobromide
- **(b)** 30 × 120 mg powders, each containing 0.5 mg of colchicine
- **(c)** 10 × 120 mg powders, each containing 2 mg of carbachol
- **(d)** 20 × 120 mg powders, each containing 0.4 mg of atropine sulphate

(e) 15 × 120 mg powders, each containing 0.2 mg of digoxin
(f) 30 × 120 mg powders, each containing 0.4 mg of atropine sulphate
(g) 20 × 120 mg powders, each containing 0.5 mg of colchicine
(h) 25 × 120 mg powders, each containing 2 mg of carbachol
(i) 20 × 120 mg powders, each containing 0.2 mg of digoxin
(j) 22 × 120 mg powders, each containing 0.5 mg of colchicine
(k) 35 × 120 mg powders, each containing 0.4 mg of atropine sulphate
(l) 28 × 120 mg powders, each containing 0.5 mg of colchicine.

9.3 Ranitidine is to be administered to a 15 kg child at 3 mg/kg twice daily for 5 days. Commercial tablets of 150 mg and 300 mg are available.

9.4 A child is to receive 1 mg loperamide daily for 3 days. A commercial tablet of 2 mg is available.

9.5 Trientine dihydrochloride is to be given to a child in a regimen of 200 mg three times a day. 18 doses are prescribed. Calculate how to prepare appropriate powders. A commercial capsule containing 300 mg is available, the contents of which weigh 318 mg.

9.6 Calculate the quantities for making 21 powders of diazoxide to be given at 2 mg/kg three times daily to a child of weight 10 kg. Capsules of 50 mg diazoxide are available.

9.7 Tretinoin 20 mg/m^2 is prescribed for a child with a body surface area of 0.3 m^2. 14 doses are being prescribed. Calculate how to prepare appropriate powders. The commercial capsule contains 10 mg of tretinoin.

For answers to these questions see page 281

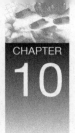

10 Suppositories and pessaries

After studying this chapter you will be able to:

- **Calibrate a suppository mould and use the mould calibration value**
- **Understand and use displacement values**
- **Determine a displacement value**
- **Calculate quantities for making suppositories and pessaries using oily bases**
- **Allow for differences occurring when using glycogelatin and other bases**

Suppositories and pessaries are made by pouring a melted base into a mould. They are, therefore, made by volume. However, both are prescribed by weight, using moulds which have a nominal capacity of 1 g, 2 g, 4 g or 8 g. The word nominal is used because they are not exactly the stated weight. Because of these limitations a number of calculations may be required to ensure that the correct dose of drug is given in each suppository.

MOULD CALIBRATION

It is necessary to calibrate a new mould in order to find out the actual capacity. This is done by making suppositories with plain base, and then weighing the suppositories produced. The calibration weight (y) is the total weight of the suppositories divided by the number of suppositories:

$$\text{Calibration weight } (y) = \frac{\text{total weight of suppositories}}{\text{number of suppositories}}$$

Example 10.1

A batch of six suppositories, of 1 g nominal weight, are produced and found to weigh 6.36 g. What is the calibration weight?

$$\text{Calibration weight } (y) = \frac{6.36}{6} = 1.06 \text{ g.}$$

Therefore the calibration weight is 1.06 g. That is, each individual suppository produced using this mould and this base will have a weight of 1.06 g.

There is a range of different bases, which may be grouped into water immiscible bases (theobroma oil, synthetic bases) and water miscible bases (glycogelatin and macrogol). Further information is available in the 3rd edition of *Pharmaceutical Practice* or the 12th edition of *The Pharmaceutical Codex*. Different bases will have slightly different calibration values, although in practice it is taken that theobroma oil and the synthetic oily bases have the same calibration weight.

DISPLACEMENT VALUES AND INCORPORATION OF A DRUG

The relative density of both the drug and the base have to be considered. If the density of the drug is the same as that of the base, then 1 g of drug will displace 1 g of base, or 1 mL of drug will displace 1 mL of base. However, in many cases there is a difference between the density of the drug and the base. This means that different amounts of base will be 'displaced', as a drug of different density is used. The higher the density of the drug, the less the volume it will displace for the same weight incorporated, because:

$$\text{Density} = \frac{\text{weight}}{\text{volume}}$$

Since the filling of the mould is by volume, a high density material will require the use of more base to fill the mould, whilst a low density material will require the use of less base. These differences are calculated by using the displacement value (DV).

Displacement value is defined as 'the number of parts by weight of drug which displaces 1 part by weight of base'. Published values of these can be found in a number of reference sources including *Pharmaceutical Practice*, *Pharmaceutical Handbook* and *The Pharmaceutical Codex* (12th edition). Sometimes, the values can vary slightly between the sources, so it is good practice to quote the source when carrying out a calculation.

To calculate the quantity of base required, a simple equation is used:

$$\text{Amount of base} = (N \times y) - \frac{N \times D}{DV}$$

where N is the number of suppositories to be made, y is the mould calibration, D is the weight (dose) of drug in one suppository and DV is the displacement value.

Before giving a worked example, there is one other piece of information required. The base will be melted, and it is not possible to completely empty the evaporating basin. Thus it is necessary to calculate for an excess of two additional suppositories.

Example 10.2

Calculate the quantities required to prepare 6 suppositories weighing 1 g, each containing 250 mg of bismuth subgallate (DV = 2.7 and mould calibration = 0.94 g).

An excess of 2 is required, therefore calculate for 8 suppositories, using the terms in the equation: $N = 8$, $y = 0.94$, $D = 250$ mg $= 0.250$ g, $DV = 2.7$. (Note conversion of drug weight into grams to match the units for the mould.)
Using the equation:

$$\text{Amount of base required} = (8 \times 0.94) - \frac{(8 \times 0.25)}{2.7} = 7.52 - 0.741$$

$$= 6.779 \text{ g} = 6.78 \text{ g}.$$

To complete the quantities for preparing the suppositories:

Bismuth subgallate $= 8 \times 0.25$ g $= 2.00$ g
Suppository base $= 6.78$ g.

Note: The quantities do not add up to 8 g because the mould calibration was not 1 g and the bismuth subgallate does not displace 2 g of base.

INCORPORATING MORE THAN ONE DRUG IN A SUPPOSITORY

Sometimes, more than one drug is required. In these situations, the equation has to be modified to allow for the displacement of each drug.

Example 10.3

Calculate the quantities required to prepare 10 suppositories each weighing 2 g and containing 150 mg of bismuth subgallate and 200 mg of zinc oxide. (Mould calibration is 2.04, DV of bismuth subgallate is 2.7, DV of zinc oxide is 4.7)

The equation is modified to:

$$\text{Amount of base} = (N \times y) - \frac{N \times D_b}{DV_b} - \frac{N \times D_z}{DV_z}$$

where N is number of suppositories, y is the mould calibration, D_b is the amount of bismuth subgallate, DV_b is the displacement value of bismuth subgallate, D_z is the amount of zinc oxide, DV_z is the displacement value of zinc oxide.

$$\text{Amount of base} = (12 \times 2.04) - \frac{(12 \times 0.15)}{2.7} - \frac{(12 \times 0.2)}{4.7}$$

$$= 24.48 - 0.667 - 0.511 = 23.30 \text{ g}$$

The final quantities required are:

Bismuth subgallate	1.80 g
Zinc oxide	2.40 g
Suppository base	23.30 g

GLYCOGELATIN AND OTHER WATER-MISCIBLE BASES

Glycogelatin is a base made of gelatin and glycerol. It can be used for pessaries and for laxative suppositories. The density of these bases is higher than that for the oily bases and so a greater weight of base is required to fill the mould. That is, a greater weight is required to produce the same volume. The figure used is called the density factor. It is 1.2 for glycogelatin base, so the mould calibration weight should be multiplied by 1.2.

In the same way, bases made using macrogols have a higher density, the density factor being taken as 1.25.

Strictly, the displacement value of drugs should also be different for these bases. However, this correction is small and it is usually assumed to make no difference. If necessary, it is possible to determine both the density factor and the revised displacement values using the methods given later in this chapter.

Example 10.4
Prepare 6 glycogelatin pessaries, of 2 g weight, each containing 500 mg of metronidazole. (DV = 1.7 and mould calibration 1.95.)

Number to make = 8. The terms in the equation will be: $N = 8$, $y = 1.95$, $D = 0.5$ g, DV = 1.7, density factor = 1.2.

$$\text{Weight of base required} = (8 \times 1.95 \times 1.2) - \frac{(8 \times 0.5)}{1.7}$$
$$= 18.72 - 2.353 = 16.37 \text{ g.}$$

Quantities required:

Metronidazole	4 g
Glycogelatin base	16.37 g

SUPPOSITORIES PRESCRIBED BY PERCENTAGE

The calculations for suppositories prescribed by percentage are simpler, because there is no need to use displacement values. Where appropriate, it is still necessary to use the density factor for the base to ensure that there is sufficient base to fill the mould.

Example 10.5
℞

Lactic acid	5%
Glycogelatin base	to 8 g
With 4 pessaries	

Assume the mould calibration value is 8.0 and the density factor is 1.2. An excess of 2 pessaries is required, therefore prepare for 6. The quantity of base required if there is no drug is $6 \times 8 \times 1.2$ g = 57.6 g. Weight of lactic acid is 5% of 57.6 g = 2.88 g. Weight of base is $57.6 - 2.88 = 54.72$ g.

Quantities required:

Lactic acid   2.88 g
Glycogelatin base   54.72 g.

DETERMINATION OF DISPLACEMENT VALUE

The displacement value can be determined for any drug by comparing the weights of plain suppositories with those containing a known concentration of the drug. To calculate the displacement value for the drug, it is necessary to prepare two batches of suppositories, one plain and the other containing a known percentage of the drug.

Example 10.6

A batch of 6 plain suppositories was prepared and found to weigh 6.3 g. Then a batch of 6 suppositories containing 20% drug was prepared and found to weigh 7.5 g.

In the medicated suppositories, the weight of the base is 80% of the total weight:

$$\text{Weight of base} = \frac{80 \times 7.5}{100} = 6.0 \text{ g.}$$

In the medicated suppositories, the weight of the drug is 20% of the total weight:

$$\text{Weight of drug} = \frac{20 \times 7.5}{100} = 1.5 \text{ g.}$$

Therefore, the weight of base displaced by the drug = 6.3 − 6.0 = 0.3 g. If 0.3 g of base is displaced by 1.5 g of the drug, then 1 g of drug will be displaced by:

$$\text{Amount of base displaced} = \frac{1.5}{0.3} = 5.$$

This figure, 5, is the displacement value of the drug.

SELF-STUDY QUESTIONS

Unless indicated to the contrary, assume that an oily base is being used and that the mould calibration is the same as the nominal mould capacity. Calculate for the number of

suppositories indicated, i.e. do not calculate for an excess.
Answer to a maximum of 2 decimal places.

10.1 Calculate the mould calibration for a batch of plain
suppositories:

(a) 6 suppositories which weigh 5.88 g
(b) 8 suppositories which weigh 8.16 g
(c) 6 suppositories which weigh 12.30 g
(d) 6 suppositories which weigh 23.93 g
(e) 12 suppositories which weigh 24.48 g.

10.2 Calculate the mould calibration for a batch of 6
suppositories which weighed 5.94 g; only 5 suppositories
were complete, which together weighed 5.05 g.

10.3 Calculate the quantity of base required to make the
following batches of suppositories:

(a) 8×1 g suppositories each containing 100 mg of aspirin
(DV 1.1)
(b) 6×1 g suppositories each containing 125 mg of
paracetamol (DV 1.5)
(c) 6×4 g suppositories each containing 500 mg of
aminophylline (DV 1.3)
(d) 8×1 g suppositories each containing 25 mg of
dimenhydrinate (DV 1.3)
(e) 6×2 g suppositories each containing 125 mg of
paracetamol (DV 1.5)
(f) 10×1 g suppositories each containing 325 mg of chloral
hydrate (DV 1.4)
(g) 10×4 g suppositories each containing 500 mg of
aminophylline (DV 1.3)
(h) 6×1 g suppositories each containing 150 mg of zinc
oxide (DV 4.7)
(i) 6×2 g suppositories each containing 500 mg of
paracetamol (DV 1.5)
(j) 6×2 g suppositories each containing 100 mg of aspirin
(DV 1.1)
(k) 8×2 g suppositories each containing 500 mg of
aminophylline (DV 1.3)

(l) 10 × 1 g suppositories each containing 150 mg of zinc oxide (DV 4.7)

(m) 10 × 2 g suppositories each containing 125 mg of paracetamol (DV 1.5)

(n) 10 × 1 g suppositories each containing 25 mg of dimenhydrinate (DV 1.3)

(o) 6 × 1 g suppositories each containing 325 mg of chloral hydrate (DV 1.4)

(p) 10 × 1 g suppositories each containing 100 mg of aspirin (DV 1.1).

10.4 Calculate the quantity of drug and base required to make each of the following:

(a) 10 × 2 g suppositories each containing 100 mg of aspirin (DV 1.1)

(b) 8 × 4 g suppositories each containing 500 mg of aminophylline (DV 1.3)

(c) 10 × 1 g suppositories each containing 125 mg of paracetamol (DV 1.5)

(d) 6 × 2 g suppositories each containing 500 mg of aminophylline (DV 1.3)

(e) 6 × 1 g suppositories each containing 100 mg of aspirin (DV 1.1)

(f) 10 × 2 g suppositories each containing 500 mg of paracetamol (DV 1.5)

(g) 8 × 1 g suppositories each containing 150 mg of zinc oxide (DV 4.7).

10.5 Calculate the quantities for twelve 1 g suppositories containing 100 mg hamamelis dry extract and zinc oxide 300 mg in a fatty base. (DV: hamamelis dry extract 1.5, zinc oxide 4.7; mould calibration: 1.0).

10.6 Calculate the quantities (drugs and base) for the following prescriptions:

(a) Six 2 g suppositories containing 200 mg hamamelis dry extract and zinc oxide 650 mg in a fatty base. (DV: hamamelis dry extract 1.5, zinc oxide 4.7; mould calibration: 1.98)

(b) Bismuth subgallate 200 mg
Resorcinol   65 mg
Zinc oxide   130 mg
Prepare 6 × 1 g suppositories (DV: bismuth subgallate 2.7, resorcinol 1.5, zinc oxide 4.7; mould calibration: 1)

(c) Bismuth subgallate   200 mg
Resorcinol   65 mg
Zinc oxide   130 mg
Prepare 6 × 1 g suppositories
(DV: bismuth subgallate 2.7, resorcinol 1.5, zinc oxide 4.7; mould calibration: 1.04)

(d) Bismuth subgallate 150 mg
Resorcinol   100 mg
Zinc oxide   100 mg
Prepare 12 × 1 g suppositories
(DV: bismuth subgallate 2.7, resorcinol 1.5, zinc oxide 4.7; mould calibration: 1)

(e) Bismuth subgallate   200 mg
Resorcinol   100 mg
Zinc oxide   250 mg
Prepare 10 × 2 g suppositories
(DV: bismuth subgallate 2.7, resorcinol 1.5, zinc oxide 4.7; mould calibration: 1.96).

10.7 How much glycogelatin base is required to prepare twelve 4 g suppositories using a mould with a calibration of 4.12?

10.8 How much macrogol base is required to prepare ten 2 g suppositories using a mould with a calibration of 2.03?

10.9 Calculate the quantities (drug and base) required to prepare the following suppositories in a macrogol base:

(a) Six 1 g suppositories containing 50 mg hydrocortisone. (DV: 1.5; mould calibration: 1.03)
(b) Ten 1 g suppositories containing 100 mg procaine hydrochloride. (DV: 1.2; mould calibration: 1.03)

(c) Six 2 g suppositories containing 50 mg tannic acid. (DV: 1.3; mould calibration: 1.93.)

10.10 What quantities are required to prepare the following products in glycogelatin base?
(a) Six 4 g pessaries containing 100 mg procaine hydrochloride. (DV: 1.2; mould calibration: 3.86)
(b) Six 2 g suppositories containing 300 mg sulfanilamide. (DV: 1.7; mould calibration: 2.12)
(c) Forty 1 g suppositories containing 0.2% castor oil. (DV: 1.0; mould calibration: 1.08).

10.11 Calculate the quantities for preparing 12 morphine sulphate suppositories containing 1% drug in a fatty base. (DV: 1.6; mould calibration: 0.98)

10.12 What quantities of glycogelatin base and lactic acid are required to prepare 10 pessaries containing 3% lactic acid? (Mould calibration: 4.12)

10.13 A prescription requires twelve 5% zinc oxide suppositories. Calculate the quantities required. (DV: 4.7; mould calibration: 0.98)

10.14 What quantities are required to prepare 60 suppositories containing 0.1% phenol? (DV: 1.1; mould calibration: 1.12)

10.15 How much base and menthol are required to make twenty 0.3% menthol in macrogol base suppositories? (DV: 0.7; mould calibration: 1.01)

10.16 During determination of the displacement value of a new drug the following information was obtained. What is the displacement value?
(a) A batch of twelve 1 g plain suppositories weighed 12.6 g and a similar batch containing 10% drug weighed 13.1 g.

(b) A batch of six 1 g plain suppositories weighed 6.28 g
and a similar batch containing 15% drug weighed
6.42 g.

(c) A batch of six 4 g plain suppositories weighed 23.76 g
and a similar batch containing 20% drug weighed
25.86 g.

(d) A batch of six 1 g plain suppositories weighed 5.94 g and
a similar batch containing 10% drug weighed 6.46 g.

For answers to these questions see page 283

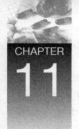

11

Calculation of doses

After studying this chapter you will be able to:

- **Understand the terms and abbreviations used when referring to dosage**
- **Calculate the numbers of tablets and capsules to fill a prescription**
- **Calculate the amount of liquid and semi-solid medicines required to fill out prescriptions**
- **Ascertain when an oral syringe is required**
- **Check the suitability of prescribed doses**
- **Calculate doses based on patient weight and body surface area**
- **Calculate doses in units and for administration by injection**

INTRODUCTION

The dosage of a drug given to a patient is important. Too little and there will be reduced therapeutic effect, too much and there could be toxicity, even death. Whilst it is the responsibility of the prescriber to decide on the dose being prescribed, the dispensing pharmacist has a key function in confirming that the dose is suitable. In many situations this is relatively straightforward, involving checking relevant reference sources. However, there are a number of situations where the processes are a little more complex.

Before proceeding it is necessary to clarify some of the terminology used. Essentially a 'dose' is the amount of drug which is taken by or administered to a patient. The 'dose' may be the amount of drug contained in a medicine, for example 300 mg of aspirin in a tablet, or it may refer to the amount of the medicine taken, for example, 1 tablet, 2 capsules, 5 mL spoonful.

Reference sources give different types of 'doses'. A few examples will be used to illustrate the terminology used.

- Single dose: this is a single administration of a drug, usually in the form of a medicine. For example, clotrimazole 500 mg pessary is used for the treatment of vaginal candidiasis as a single application at night.
- Daily dose: this is the amount of drug recommended to be used in one day. For example, the *British National Formulary* indicates that for atorvastatin the dose is usually 10 mg once daily (for primary and combined hypercholesterolaemia).
- Daily divided dose: this is where a total amount of drug per day is specified, with the recommendation that it should be administered on several occasions during the day. For example, lorazepam for anxiety has an oral dose of 1–4 mg daily in divided doses, whilst for insomnia associated with anxiety a single dose of 1–2 mg at bedtime is recommended. The doses for the elderly and children are also different.
- Weekly dose: this is where infrequent dosage is used. Methotrexate is used for treating psoriasis, the oral dose being given as 10–25 mg once weekly.
- Total dose: this is where a drug may be administered continuously or intermittently up to a maximum total amount. For example, 2.5 mg of atenolol is given by intravenous injection for arrhythmias at a rate of 1 mg/min, repeated at 5-minute intervals to a maximum of 10 mg atenolol.
- Dose range: this is the term used to denote that a drug is normally used over a range of different doses. The doses for lorazepam given above are examples of this.

The examples used above indicate that doses appear in many different forms and this can lead to some complications in the interpretation of dosage information. There are other variations to those given above; for example, where a repeat dosage is permitted or where the dosages are different for different disease states. The response of the patient may also influence the dose, as for example in asthma, diabetes and anticoagulant therapy.

A dosage regimen is scheduling of the administration of doses through time. For example, a daily divided dose may be taken two, three or four times in a day, or may be spaced out by time (four hourly) or may be related to meal times (before food) or to other events during the day (bedtime, before breakfast). In other situations, doses may be spaced out over longer time spans. For example, some steroids may be used on alternate days, whilst many of the cytotoxic drugs are given at well-spaced intervals to minimize toxicity.

In this chapter a number of aspects will be dealt with. The first is in situations where the pharmacist has to calculate the amount of medicine or number of unit dosage forms required. These are usually simple calculations involving working out how many tablets or capsules, or how much liquid medicine, to supply to the patient. Then problems involved in checking for the suitability of a prescribed dose will be considered. Finally, calculations to determine how much drug is to be supplied for the patient will be demonstrated.

There are special considerations surrounding paediatric doses which will be dealt with in Chapter 12. There are also some dose-related issues arising with intravenous additives and infusion rate calculations which are dealt with in Chapter 14.

AMOUNT OF MEDICINE REQUIRED FOR A PRESCRIPTION

Solid dosage forms

Tablets and capsules are manufactured in fixed strengths. Sometimes, only one strength is available, whereas in other cases several different strengths are manufactured. Whilst it is desirable that the prescriber specifies the number of tablets or capsules required, this is not always the case. Prescribers may specify the dose and the frequency at which they are to be administered and the duration of the treatment. In these situations the pharmacist must calculate the number of individual tablets or capsules to supply to the patient. A number of different examples follow.

Example 11.1

The doctor prescribes levodopa, 500 mg to be taken every 8 hours for 28 days. Levodopa is available as 500 mg tablets. How many tablets should be supplied?

For each dose, 1 tablet is required.
A frequency of 'every eight hours' means that there are 3 doses per day.
Therefore, the total number of tablets required is $1 \times 3 \times 28 = 84$ tablets.

Example 11.2

Calculate the number of tablets to be dispensed when the prescription states: One tablet twice daily 2/52.

Frequently doctors will use abbreviations for time spans. Common abbreviations are shown in Table 11.1. From this it can be seen that /52 indicates 'weeks', and therefore 2/52 is two weeks.
Therefore, two tablets are to be taken daily for 14 days = $2 \times 14 = 28$ tablets.

Example 11.3

How many tablets should be provided when the prescription specifies two tablets to be taken four times daily for 3/52?

There will be $2 \times 4 = 8$ tablets each day.
3/52 indicates three weeks, that is 21 days.
Number of tablets required is $21 \times 8 = 168$ tablets.

Table 11.1   Commonly used abbreviations for durations used on prescriptions (including the indication of age).

Abbreviation	Meaning	Example	Interpretation of example
d	day	7d	7 days
/24	hour	6/24	6 hours
/7	day	5/7	5 days
/52	week	3/52	3 weeks
		4/52	1 month
/12*	month	7/12	7 months

* Often used when indicating the age of a baby.

Example 11.4

A prescription requires 50 mg of dipyridamole four times daily for a month. Dipyridamole is available as 25 mg and 100 mg tablets. How many tablets should be dispensed?

There is no tablet of the required dosage, therefore two 25 mg tablets will be used.

These will be taken four times daily, therefore the daily need is $4 \times 2 = 8$ tablets.

Supply for 1 month is requested. This is taken to be 28 days.

Therefore total number of tablets required is $8 \times 28 = 224$ tablets.

Example 11.5

A prescription requires 150 mg of dipyridamole four times daily for a month. Dipyridamole is available as 25 mg and 100 mg tablets. How many of which tablets should be dispensed?

Whilst it would be possible for the patient to take 6 tablets on each occasion, it is better to use a combination of two different strengths of tablet.

Thus the 100 mg tablet can be used, the number required being $4 \times 28 = 112$ of the 100 mg tablets.

The 25 mg tablets will have to be used to provide the additional 50 mg, that is 2 tablets at each dose time. The number of 25 mg tablets required is $2 \times 4 \times 28 = 224$ of the 25 mg tablets.

The patient will be instructed to take one 100 mg tablet and two 25 mg tablets four times a day.

Example 11.6

A patient requires to take 5 mg prednisolone tablets following a tapering dose regimen: 25 mg for 3 days, then reducing by 5 mg every 3 days until the course is finished. How many 5 mg tablets should be supplied?

This 'tailing off' is normal practice with steroids. To answer the question, it is necessary to work out the dose regimen logically. For each dosage period, the individual number of tablets can be calculated.

25 mg for 3 days; 5 tablets for 3 days = 15 tablets
20 mg for 3 days; 4 tablets for 3 days = 12 tablets
15 mg for 3 days; 3 tablets for 3 days = 9 tablets
10 mg for 3 days; 2 tablets for 3 days = 6 tablets
5 mg for 3 days; 1 tablet for 3 days = 3 tablets

The number of tablets can now be totalled = $15 + 12 + 9 + 6 + 3 = 45$ tablets

Example 11.7

A patient receives a prescription for an antibiotic with the instruction to take two capsules at first and then one every six hours. The doctor specifies 29 capsules. How long will the treatment last?

A dose regimen of 'every six hours' indicates 4 capsules per day. The duration of the regimen is 29/4 = 7 days, plus one additional capsule. However, the initial dose is of two capsules, therefore the regimen will last exactly 7 days.

Example 11.8

A doctor writes a prescription for a patient to take 3.5 g of ispaghula husk twice daily for ten days. Ispaghula husk is available commercially as Fybogel® and Ispagel® in 3.5 g sachets. How is the prescription to be dispensed?

Either of the two commercial products will provide the required dose. Two sachets are required each day, for 10 days, therefore 20 sachets should be dispensed.

Liquids

Example 11.9

Ranitidine oral solution contains 75 mg/5 mL. How many milligrams of ranitidine are contained in 10 mL, 15 mL, 25 mL?

All these doses are multiples of 5 mL, so it is a simple matter of multiplication. However, if intermediate volumes were specified, simple proportion would be used. To illustrate this, doses will be calculated using simple proportion. Let the dose (in milligrams) be y in each case:

For 10 mL, $\dfrac{10}{5} = \dfrac{y}{75}$, therefore $y = \dfrac{10 \times 75}{5} = 150$ mg/10 mL

For 15 mL, $\dfrac{15}{5} = \dfrac{y}{75}$, therefore $y = \dfrac{15 \times 75}{5} = 225$ mg/15 mL

For 25 mL, $\dfrac{25}{5} = \dfrac{y}{75}$, therefore $y = \dfrac{25 \times 75}{5} = 375$ mg/25 mL

Example 11.10

What is the total volume to be dispensed when the prescription states: '5 mL twice daily for 3/52'?

3/52 means 3 weeks, 21 days.
Therefore, the amount to be dispensed is $5 \times 2 \times 21 = 210$ mL.

Example 11.11

Calculate the volume of each dose and the total quantity to be dispensed to fill a prescription for paracetamol suspension, with the instructions '500 mg, four times daily for 14d'. A commercial paracetamol suspension is available containing 250 mg/5 mL.

Since there is a dose of 250 mg in 5 mL and a dose of 500 mg is required, the volume required will be 10 mL per dose.
Therefore there will be 10×4 mL per day = 40 mL; 14 days (14d) will require $14 \times 40 = 560$ mL.

Example 11.12

The following prescription is received: sodium valproate oral solution, 100 mg to be given twice daily for 2 weeks.

Sodium valproate oral solution contains sodium valproate 200 mg/5 mL. This prescription is therefore translated as: 2.5 mL to be given twice daily for 2 weeks.
The quantity to be dispensed will be:

$$2.5 \times 2 \times 14 = 70 \text{ mL}$$

The dose of solution required, 2.5 mL, may only be measured using an oral syringe (see over).

Example 11.13

A prescription is written for 200 mL of a suspension containing 30 mg/5 mL and instruction to take 60 mg twice daily. How many days' supply does this prescription contain?

60 mg is contained in 10 mL, therefore 20 mL will be taken each day. With a total of 200 mL, this represents 10 days' supply.

Example 11.14

A patient is to take a 120 mg dose from a 2.4% w/v suspension three times per day. What volume should be taken and how much should be dispensed to provide sufficient quantity for 14 days?

Calculate the volume containing 120 mg.
A 2.4% w/v suspension contains 2400 mg in 100 mL, therefore it will contain:

$$120 \text{ mg in } \frac{100 \times 120}{2400} = 5 \text{ mL}$$

Therefore, each dose will be 5 mL. The total volume required is $5 \times 3 \times 14 = 210$ mL.

Oral syringes

If fractional doses are prescribed for oral liquids, they should not be diluted, but an oral syringe should be supplied with the dispensed oral liquid. The standard oral syringe is marked in 0.5 mL divisions from 1 to 5 mL to measure doses of less than 5 mL. An adapter fits into the neck of all common sizes of the medicine bottle. Instructions should be supplied with the oral syringe. Further information is included in the 3rd edition of *Pharmaceutical Practice*.

External preparations

There are fewer calculations concerning doses and quantities of medicine required with external products. However, there are occasions when the prescriber omits the total quantity and the guidance included in the *British National Formulary* (BNF) may be required. Table 11.2 presents the quantities considered suitable in the BNF for dermatological preparations for different parts of the body.

Table 11.2 Suitable quantities of dermatological preparations as given in the BNF. The quantities are for an adult, applying twice daily for 1 week.

Body site	Cream or ointment	Lotion	Corticosteroid cream or ointment
Face	15–30 g	100 mL	–
Face and neck	–	–	15–30 g
Both hands	25–50 g	200 mL	15–30 g
Scalp	50–100 g	200 mL	15–30 g
Both arms	100–200 g	200 mL	30–60 g
Both legs	100–200 g	200 mL	100 g
Trunk	400 g	500 mL	100 g
Groin and genitalia	15–25 g	100 mL	15–30 g

Example 11.15
A patient is prescribed 1% hydrocortisone ointment to be applied to the right arm, three times daily for 2 weeks. How much ointment should be supplied?

Hydrocortisone is a corticosteroid.

Table 11.2 specifies that both arms would require 30–60 g for twice daily application over 1 week. Therefore, for one arm, we require 15–30 g over the same dose regimen. For the three times daily frequency and two weeks' duration, we require:

$$\frac{15 \times 3 \times 2}{2} = 45 \text{ g, and } \frac{30 \times 3 \times 2}{2} = 90 \text{ g.}$$

Note: The ointment will be pre-manufactured and so will be dispensed in predetermined sizes of tubes. At the time of writing, the BNF only lists a 15 g tube of 1% hydrocortisone. Depending on the size of the individual, four 15 g tubes is probably a reasonable amount to supply.

SUITABILITY OF DOSES

An important function of the pharmacist is to check that the dose of a drug prescribed for a patient is appropriate. Potential problems arise due to variation in terminology used in expressing the dosage. Be alert, because a lack of awareness could have very serious consequences.

Example 11.16

The following prescription is received:

℞

Verapamil tablets   160 milligrams
Send 56
Take two tablets twice daily

There are a variety of doses quoted for verapamil in the BNF depending on the condition being treated. They are as follows for oral administration (there is also a dose for slow intravenous injection):
Supraventricular arrhythmias, 40–120 mg three times daily.
Angina, 80–120 mg three times daily.
Hypertension, 240–480 mg daily in 2–3 divided doses.
The dose given for hypertension is stated in a significantly different way. Whereas the doses for the other two conditions can be given three times daily, indicating a maximum of 360 mg in any one day, the hypertension dose is stated as the total dose to be given in any one day and is divided up and given at the stated frequencies (daily divided dose), i.e. a maximum of 240 mg, given twice daily or a maximum of 160 mg, given three times daily.

The prescription is for a dose of $160 \times 2 = 320$ mg to be taken twice a day. Thus, the prescribed dose is higher than recommended in the BNF, so consultation with the prescriber would be required.

Example 11.17

A prescription for Ranitidine Oral Solution is received, with a dose regimen of two 5-mL spoonfuls, three times daily.

The BNF indicates that ranitidine oral solution provides a dose of 75 mg/5 mL. In the same source we find that there are different dosages given for ranitidine depending on the condition being treated and the progress in the management of the disease. Thus, for benign gastric and duodenal ulceration 150 mg can be given twice daily, or 300 mg given at night, and there are also recommendations for duration of treatment. Further, in cases of NSAID-associated duodenal ulceration 300 mg can be given twice daily for 4 weeks to achieve a higher healing rate.

Thus the highest dosage rate is 600 mg per day in the latter case. The prescription is requesting 75×2 mg = 150 mg three times a day, that is a total of 450 mg daily.

Thus there are two issues. Firstly, is the patient suffering from an NSAID-related duodenal ulcer? Secondly, the frequency of dosage is unusual. This dosage and frequency can be used in the Zollinger–Ellison syndrome, although a proton pump inhibitor is preferred. It would be advisable to confirm the intentions of the prescriber before dispensing this prescription.

Doses based on patient's weight

The doses which have been discussed so far in this chapter have been for drugs which have a relatively wide therapeutic range, in other words where an accurate control of dosage is not critical. As the therapeutic range narrows, so it becomes more important that the dose is related to the individual patient. For some drugs the amount of drug has to be calculated accurately for the particular patient. This is normally carried out using either body weight or body surface area. When body weight is used, the dose will be expressed as mg/kg. In countries which still use pounds, it will be necessary to convert the patient's weight in pounds into kilograms by dividing by 2.2 (see Ch. 2).

The weight of patients being prescribed these drugs should be known. However, there may be situations where the weight of the patient is unknown. There are tables giving 'desirable' weights depending on height and size of body frame (small, medium or large build) and for men and women separately (for example *Pharmaceutical Handbook*). These may provide a useful guide. An alternative figure which can be obtained is the 'ideal body weight'. This figure is used in calculating the creatinine clearance rate (see Ch. 17) and is calculated from the height of the patient using a range of equations depending on age and height. For adults (over 18 years), the equations are as follows:

Male:

Ideal body weight (kg) = 50 + (2.3 × inches over 5 feet)

Female:

Ideal body weight (kg) = 45.5 + (2.3 × inches over 5 feet)

The BNF gives the ideal body weight of an adult male as 68 kg and an adult female as 56 kg.

When a drug is prescribed as a dose per kilogram, the actual quantity to be administered is obtained by multiplying the weight (in kg) of the patient by the dose per kilogram.

Example 11.18
What dose of procainamide should be given to a patient weighing 71 kg to provide an intravenous infusion dose of 700 µg/kg per minute?

The dose required is 700 × 71 = 49700 µg = 49.7 mg per minute.

Example 11.19
A patient, weighing 165 lb, is to receive an intramuscular injection of tobramycin, 4 mg/kg. How much tobramycin is required?

The patient's weight is in pounds and the dose in kilograms, so the patient's weight is divided by 2.2 to convert it to kilograms:

Patient's weight = 165/2.2 = 75 kg

The dose of tobramycin required = 75 × 4 = 300 mg.

Example 11.20
A prescription is received for two intramuscular injections of gentamicin giving a 300 mg dose of gentamicin at 12 hourly intervals. Comment on the prescription. (The patient weighs 70 kg)

The BNF indicates that the dose range for gentamicin by intramuscular injection is '3–5 mg/kg daily (in divided doses every 8 hours)'. In order to be able to comment on the suitability of this prescription, it is necessary to convert the dose prescribed into a dose/kg.

The dose per kilogram = 300/70 = 4.29 mg/kg

It can be seen that this is towards the top end of the range. However, the BNF indicates that this range should be given in divided doses, at 8 hourly intervals. Therefore the prescribed dose is too high. Also, this dose is to be repeated after 12 hours, increasing the daily dose to well in excess of the maximum dosage in the BNF. There would also need to be a good reason for decreasing the frequency of dosage, because this could cause plasma concentrations of the gentamicin to fall below therapeutic levels.

Doses based on surface area

Body surface area is a more accurate method for calculating doses and is used where extreme accuracy is required. This is necessary where there is a very narrow range of plasma concentration between the desired therapeutic effect and severe toxicity, such as with drugs used to treat cancer. The average body surface area of a 70 kg adult is about 1.8 m². The body surface area can be calculated from body weight and height using one of the equations given below. The use of a nomogram for calculating body surface area in children is dealt with in Chapter 12.

Body surface area (m²) = weight (kg)$^{0.425}$ + height (cm)$^{0.725}$ × 0.007184

Body surface area (m²) = (height (inches) × weight (pounds)/3131)$^{1/2}$

Body surface area (m²) = (height (centimetres) × weight (kg) /3600)$^{1/2}$

Example 11.21

A patient is to receive 40 mg/m² daunorubicin intravenously. The patient has a body surface area of 1.90 m². What weight of daunorubicin is required?

This is a straightforward multiplication: 40 × 1.9 = 76 mg daunorubicin.

Example 11.22

A patient is 170 cm tall and weighs 78 kg. He is to receive 1.8 mg/m² vincristine. How much vincristine should be included in the injection?

The first step is to calculate the body surface area. The weight and height are in metric units, so the third form of the equation opposite can be used:

Body surface area (m²) = (height (centimetres) × weight (kg) /3600)¹ᐟ².

Substituting: body surface area =
$(170 \times 78/3600)^{1/2} = \sqrt{3.683} = 1.919$ m².

The dose of drug can now be calculated = 1.919 × 1.8 = 3.45 mg
vincristine.

Example 11.23

A prescription is received for fifteen 100 mg etoposide capsules, three to be taken daily for five days. The lady is 5 feet 5 inches tall and weighs 8 stones 8 pounds.

Reference to the BNF shows that oral etoposide is used at a dose range of 120–240 mg/m² daily for 5 days. Therefore, the body surface area must be calculated. The patient's height is 65 inches and weight is 120 pounds.

Body surface area (m²) = (height (inches) × weight (pounds)/3131)¹ᐟ²

Substituting: body surface area = $(65 \times 120/3131)^{1/2} = 1.58$ m²

It is now possible to calculate the recommended dose range of etoposide for this patient: 1.58 × 120 = 190 mg to
1.58 × 240 = 379 mg daily for five days.
The prescribed daily dose of 300 mg is within this range and so appears to be acceptable.

Doses involving units

As described in Chapter 2, units are used for large molecule drugs of biological origin when potency may vary from one batch to another. Dosage calculations involving units are essentially the same as with any other drug.

Example 11.24

A patient is to receive 1.5 million units of oral colistin every eight hours for one week for bowel sterilization. Colistin is available as tablets (1.5 million units per tablet) or a syrup (containing 250 000 units per 5 mL). What quantities of tablets or syrup would be required?

Checking with the BNF confirms that the dose is in the normal range.
Tablets: Each dose is one tablet, 3 times a day for 7
days = $1 \times 3 \times 7$ = 21 tablets.
Syrup: Each dose requires 6×5 mL spoonfuls, 3 times a day for 7
days = $30 \times 3 \times 7$ = 630 mL, with instructions to take six 5-mL
spoonfuls every eight hours.

INTRAVENOUS INJECTION DOSES

Some of the examples used earlier in this chapter were for
injections. For an injection a syringe has to be used into
which is drawn the correct amount of solution to provide the
required dose. The accuracy to which volumes can be
measured in syringes depends on the size of the syringe—
and therefore on the volume being measured. Syringes of
greater than 1 mL capacity, for example 3 mL and 6 mL, have
graduations at 0.1 mL intervals. Therefore, it is not possible to
measure any more accurately than to the nearest 0.1 mL. The
answer to any calculations where the volume is greater than
1 mL should only be calculated to the first decimal place.
Syringes with a capacity of 1 mL or less are usually calibrated
in hundredths of a millilitre, that is 0.01 mL graduations.
Therefore, the answer to any calculations where the volume is
less than 1 mL should be calculated to the second decimal
place.

Example 11.25
A patient is prescribed an injection of 65 mg of pethidine. Stock
ampoules of pethidine contain 100 mg in 2 mL. Calculate the volume
of the injection.

The calculation is carried out by simple proportion. Let the required
volume be y mL:

$$\text{Therefore } \frac{y}{65} = \frac{2}{100}, \text{ therefore } y = \frac{2 \times 65}{100} = 1.3 \text{ mL}$$

The volume is larger than 1 mL, therefore the accuracy of 1 decimal
place only is needed.

Example 11.26

Morphine 5.5 mg is prescribed for a patient. The stock ampoule contains 10 mg/mL. What volume of this solution is required?

Let the required volume be y mL. By simple proportion:

$$\frac{y}{5.5} = \frac{1}{10}, \text{ therefore } y = \frac{1 \times 5.5}{10} = 0.55 \text{ mL.}$$

Here the required volume is less than 1 mL and so the figure should be accurate to the second decimal place.

Example 11.27

An injection of 450 mg of benzylpenicillin is prescribed using a stock ampoule which contains 600 mg per 5 mL. What volume should be used for the injection?

Let the required volume be y mL. By simple proportion therefore:

$$\frac{y}{450} = \frac{5}{600}, \text{ therefore } y = \frac{5 \times 450}{600} = 3.75 \text{ mL.}$$

The volume is greater than 1 mL and therefore will be administered using a syringe calibrated to 0.1 mL. The required volume must be rounded—in this case upwards—so the required volume is 3.8 mL.

SELF-STUDY QUESTIONS

Assume that 1 month is 28 days. Do not work to more than 2 decimal places and where the answer is in mg, give it to the nearest 1 mg.

11.1 Calculate the number of tablets to be dispensed when the prescription states:

(a) 1 tablet twice daily for 1/52
(b) 2 tablets twice daily for 2/52
(c) 1 tablet four times daily for 3/52
(d) 2 tablets four times daily for 2/52
(e) 1 tablet every eight hours for 1/52
(f) 1 tablet every six hours for 2/52
(g) 2 tablets every eight hours for 3/52
(h) 2 tablets every six hours for 3/52.

11.2 Specify the number and strength of tablets to be dispensed when the prescription states the following:

(a) 500 mg every six hours for 1/52. Available tablets are 125 mg and 500 mg

(b) 100 mg twice daily for 2/52. Available tablets are 50 mg and 250 mg

(c) 150 mg four times daily for 2/52. Available tablets are 50 mg and 200 mg

(d) 75 mg every eight hours for 3/52. Available tablets are 25 mg and 100 mg

(e) 200 mg twice daily for 1/12. Available tablets are 100 mg and 250 mg

(f) 250 mg twice daily for 3/52. Available tablets are 50 mg and 200 mg

(g) 150 mg twice daily for 1/12. Available tablets are 50 mg, 100 mg and 200 mg

(h) 250 mg four times daily for 3/52. Available tablets are 50 mg, 100 mg and 500 mg

(i) 25 mg every eight hours for 2/52. Available tablets are 2 mg, 5 mg and 10 mg

(j) 8 mg every eight hours for 1/12. Available tablets are 1 mg, 2 mg, 5 mg and 10 mg.

11.3 Calculate the number of days supplied when the prescription states:

(a) 84 tablets, two tablets to be taken twice daily

(b) 28 tablets, one tablet to be taken every six hours

(c) 112 tablets, one tablet to be taken four times daily

(d) 84 tablets, two tablets to be taken every eight hours

(e) 28 tablets, two tablets to be taken twice daily

(f) 112 tablets, two tablets to be taken every six hours.

11.4 How many tablets are required?

(a) Tailing off from taking prednisolone is to be carried out using 5 mg tablets, starting at 30 mg and reducing by 5 mg every 5 days.

(b) Methylprednisolone is available as a 4 mg tablet. A patient is being withdrawn, starting with a dose of 20 mg and reducing by 4 mg every 4 days.

(c) A patient is being withdrawn from taking prednisolone enteric-coated tablets. Using 2.5 mg tablets, the initial dose of 30 mg is reduced by 5 mg every 4 days.

11.5 Calculate the total volume to be dispensed when the prescription states:

(a) 5 mL twice daily for 7d
(b) 5 mL twice daily for 28d
(c) 5 mL three times daily for 2/52
(d) 5 mL twelve hourly for 3/52
(e) 5 mL three times daily for 10d
(f) 10 mL twice daily for 14d
(g) 10 mL every eight hours for 1/52
(h) 10 mL every six hours for 1/12.

11.6 How much should be dispensed for the following?

(a) 100 mg twice daily for 10d. The available medicine has 50 mg/5 mL.
(b) 50 mg every six hours for 7d. The available medicine has 25 mg/5 mL.
(c) 75 mg three times daily for 2/52. The available medicine has 25 mg/5 mL.

11.7 What is the total volume to be dispensed and the individual dose when the prescription states the following?

(a) 20 mg three times daily for 28d. The available medicine has 10 mg/mL.
(b) 50 mg twice daily for 7d. The available medicine has 100 mg/5 mL.
(c) 100 mg twice daily for 3/52. The available medicine has 250 mg/5 mL.

11.8 What is the individual dose and the total volume to be dispensed when the prescription states the following?

(a) 200 mg twice daily for 2/52. The available medicine is a 2.0% w/v suspension.
(b) 75 mg twice daily for 14d. The available medicine is a 1.5% w/v suspension.
(c) 240 mg three times daily for 2/52. The available medicine is a 1.6% w/v suspension.
(d) 250 mg three times daily for 1/52. The available medicine is a 2.5% w/v suspension.
(e) 120 mg every eight hours for 10d. The available medicine is a 2.4% w/v suspension.
(f) 120 mg six hourly for 21d. The available medicine is a 1.2% w/v suspension.

11.9 Calculate the number of days supplied when the prescription states:

(a) 5 mL twice daily and 70 mL are supplied
(b) 10 mL eight hourly and 840 mL are supplied
(c) 5 mL six hourly and 420 mL are supplied
(d) 5 mL three times daily and 210 mL are supplied
(e) 10 mL twice daily and 280 mL are supplied
(f) 5 mL three times daily and 315 mL are supplied.

11.10 Methadone oral concentrate is available as 20 mg/mL. What volume is required to provide 2 mg, 17 mg, 43 mg?

11.11 Trazodone hydrochloride liquid contains 50 mg/5 mL. What quantity of drug is contained in 1 mL, 8 mL, 20 mL?

11.12 Biphasic insulin lispro is produced as a 100 unit/mL injection in a 5 mL ampoule. What volume is required to provide a patient with 8 units? How many doses are contained in the ampoule?

11.13 Specify the quantity to be dispensed when the prescription requests a lotion to be used on the face, three times daily for 2 weeks.

11.14   An emollient is required to be applied to the trunk four times daily. Suggest a quantity for 3 weeks' treatment.

11.15   Betnovate® cream (a corticosteroid) is prescribed for application to the left leg twice daily for 2 weeks. How much cream should be prescribed?

11.16   A dandruff lotion is to be applied daily to the scalp for 2 weeks. How much lotion is required?

11.17   Dermovate® ointment (a corticosteroid) is to be applied sparingly to both hands once daily for 4 weeks. The doctor has requested a 100 g tube. Is this a reasonable quantity?

11.18   What dose of procainamide is required to provide 50 mg/kg for each of the following patients?

(a) A patient weighing 57 kg
(b) A patient weighing 81 kg
(c) A patient weighing 62 kg
(d) A patient weighing 152 pounds
(e) A patient weighing 130 pounds

11.19   What dose of atenolol should be given to a patient to provide a dose of 150 µg/kg?

(a) A patient weighing 75 kg
(b) A patient weighing 87 kg
(c) A patient weighing 81 kg
(d) A patient weighing 65 kg
(e) A patient weighing 180 pounds
(f) A patient weighing 118 pounds
(g) A patient weighing 146 pounds
(h) A patient weighing 285 pounds

11.20   Calculate the dose of zidovudine required to provide 120 mg/m^2 for each patient:

(a) A patient of estimated surface area 0.32 m^2
(b) A patient of estimated surface area 1.64 m^2

(c) A patient of estimated surface area 1.86 m^2

(d) A patient of estimated surface area 1.58 m^2

11.21 What dose of drug is required for each of the following situations?

(a) Somatropin to provide 21 units/m^2 for a patient of estimated surface area 1.74 m^2

(b) Somatropin to provide 21 units/m^2 for a patient of estimated surface area 1.96 m^2

(c) Cisplatin to provide 60 mg/m^2 for a patient of estimated surface area 1.57 m^2

(d) Cisplatin to provide 60 mg/m^2 for a patient of estimated surface area 1.68 m^2

(e) Daunorubicin to provide 25 mg/m^2 for a patient of estimated surface area 1.75 m^2

(f) Daunorubicin to provide 25 mg/m^2 for a patient of estimated surface area 1.67 m^2

11.22 What dose of drug is required for each of the following situations?

(a) Zidovudine to provide 120 mg/m^2 for a patient of height 140 cm and weight 30 kg

(b) Daunorubicin to provide 25 mg/m^2 for a patient of height 163 cm and weight 56 kg

(c) Somatropin to provide 21 units/m^2 for a patient of height 182 cm and weight 76 kg

(d) Zidovudine to provide 120 mg/m^2 for a patient of height 150 cm and weight 35 kg

(e) Somatropin to provide 21 units/m^2 for a patient of height 68 inches and weight 168 pounds

(f) Daunorubicin to provide 25 mg/m^2 for a patient of height 68 inches and weight 154 pounds

(g) Cisplatin to provide 60 mg/m^2 for a patient of height 5 feet 6 inches and weight 10 stones 3 pounds

(h) Cisplatin to provide 60 mg/m^2 for a patient of height 71 inches and weight 73 kg

(i) Cisplatin to provide 60 mg/m^2 for a patient of height 175 cm and weight 156 pounds

11.23 How many capsules should the patient take for bexarotene 300 mg/m^2? The patient has an estimated body surface area of 1.75 m^2. 75 mg capsules are available.

11.24 Indicate a suitable dosage for a patient prescribed 10 g/m^2 of sodium phenylbutyrate in three divided doses. The drug is available as 500 mg tablets. The patient has a body surface area of 1.75 m^2.

11.25 How many tablets are required to provide a patient (body surface area 1.78 m^2) with tretinoin 22.5 mg/m^2 twice daily for 1 week? Tretinoin is available as 10 mg tablets.

11.26 Calculate a suitable dosage regimen for a patient weighing 76 kg and 171 cm in height who is to receive temozolomide 200 mg/m^2 daily. Temozolomide is available as 5 mg, 20 mg and 100 mg capsules.

11.27 A patient is to receive tioguanine at a maintenance dose of 60 mg/m^2 twice daily for 14 days. How many 40 mg scored tablets should be provided and what dosage instructions should be given to the patient who has an estimated body surface area of 1.67 m^2?

11.28 An injection of amphotericin contains 50 mg/10 mL. What volume is required to provide the following?

(a) A 10 mg dose
(b) A 10.5 mg dose
(c) A 14 mg dose
(d) A 16.5 mg dose
(e) A 20 mg dose

11.29 A polymyxin E injection contains 500 000 units/mL. What volume is required to provide the following?

(a) An infusion containing 150 000 units
(b) An infusion containing 120 000 units
(c) An infusion containing 172 500 units

11.30   What volume of injection is required to provide the specified dose?

(a) Prochlorperazine 12.5 mg/mL injection to give a dose of 25 mg

(b) Protamine sulphate injection contains 50 mg/5 mL to provide a dose of 15 mg

(c) Piroxicam injection (20 mg/mL) to provide a dose of 30 mg by deep intramuscular injection

(d) Clonidine hydrochloride injection contains 300 μg per 2 mL to be added to a slow infusion to provide a dose of 750 μg over 24 hours

(e) Isosorbide dinitrate 0.05% w/v injection to provide a dose of 15 mg

(f) Amiodarone hydrochloride 150 mg/3 mL injection to provide a dose of 5 mg/kg to patient weighing 75 kg

For answers to these questions see page 285

Paediatric doses

After studying this chapter you will be able to:

- **Use equations which approximate a child's dose as a proportion of the adult dose**
- **Calculate doses based on body weight**
- **Use a nomogram to determine body surface area from the child's height and weight**
- **Calculate doses for children based on body surface area**

INTRODUCTION

Children often require different doses from those of adults. This arises for a number of reasons, including differences in the ability of children to absorb, distribute, metabolize and eliminate drugs compared to adults. It is also known that the relationships of these factors changes with the stage of development of a child. Ideally, therefore, the dose of a drug to be administered to a child should be arrived at as a result of extensive clinical studies. Frequently this is not possible and so an alternative method has to be used. Normally this is achieved by making an estimate of the children's dose from the adult dose. The methods to be discussed in this chapter include the use of age, body weight and body surface area. The most reliable method uses the body surface area and so is preferred for the most potent drugs.

In the BNF, children's doses are given under the individual monograph. Where the dose varies with age, the following age ranges and general terms are used:

1 month of life   (Neonate)
up to 1 year old   (Infant)

1–5 years
6–12 years

The term 'child' refers to any person under the age of 12 years. Anyone older than this is treated as an adult for dosage purposes.

CHILDREN'S DOSES CALCULATED BY AGE FROM THE ADULT DOSE

This method is not very sensitive and so should only be used for drugs which have a wide margin between the therapeutic and toxic doses, i.e. a wide therapeutic window. Table 12.1 is taken from the BNF and indicates the percentage of the adult dose which should be administered to children of different ages. In addition a number of formulae have been proposed to calculate the proportion of adult dose which is appropriate, using different characteristics of the child.

Table 12.1 The relationship between age, ideal body weight, height, body surface area and percentage of adult dose (after the BNF)

Age	Ideal body weight		Height		Body surface area	Percentage of adult dose*
	kg	lb	cm	in	(m²)	
Newborn	3.5	7.7	50	20	0.23	12.5
1 month	4.2	9	55	22	0.26	14.5
3 months	5.6	12	59	23	0.32	18
6 months	7.7	17	67	26	0.40	22
1 year	10	22	76	30	0.47	25
3 years	15	33	94	37	0.62	33
5 years	18	40	108	42	0.73	40
7 years	23	51	120	47	0.88	50
12 years	39	86	148	58	1.25	75

* This column is no longer included in the BNF.
Note that for the first 3 months, a pre-term infant may need a reduced dosage depending on their clinical condition.

Fried's rule (for infants younger than 1 year):

$$\text{Dose for infant} = \frac{\text{age (months)} \times \text{adult dose}}{150}$$

Young's rule:

$$\text{Dose for child} = \frac{\text{age (years)} \times \text{adult dose}}{\text{age} + 12}$$

Clark's rule:

$$\text{Dose for child} = \frac{\text{weight (in kg)} \times \text{adult dose}}{75}$$
$$= \frac{\text{weight (in lb)} \times \text{adult dose}}{150}$$

Body surface area method (BSA):

$$\text{Dose for child} = \frac{\text{BSA of child (m}^2) \times \text{adult dose}}{1.73 \text{ m}^2 \text{ (average adult BSA)}}$$

Note: Another version of this equation uses 1.80 as the denominator. The BNF indicates that the surface area of an adult male is 1.80 m^2 and an adult female is 1.60 m^2.

Example 12.1

A child of 5 years of age is prescribed a drug, the adult dose of which is 250 mg. Assuming that the child has normal values for weight, height and surface area, calculate the dose using the different methods outlined above.

Young's rule:

$$\text{Dose} = \frac{5 \times 250}{(5 + 12)} = 73.5 \text{ mg.}$$

Clark's rule:

$$\text{Dose} = \frac{18 \times 250}{75} = 60 \text{ mg (using weight in kg).}$$
$$\text{Dose} = \frac{40 \times 250}{150} = 66.7 \text{ mg (using weight in pounds).}$$

Body surface area method:

$$\text{Dose} = \frac{0.73 \times 250}{1.73} = 105.5 \text{ mg.}$$

Using the figure of 1.80 for adult body surface area, the answer becomes 101.4 mg.

Percentage method:
Table 12.1 indicates a dose of 40% of adult dose:

$$= \frac{250 \times 40}{100} = 100 \text{ mg.}$$

This simple set of calculations indicates a wide range of suggested doses for this unidentified drug. If the drug were flucloxacillin, where the adult dose is 250–500 mg, the recommended dose for a child 2–10 years in the BNF is one half of the adult dose, namely 125–250 mg. However, if it were cycloserine, the adult dose is 250 mg and the recommended child's dose is 10 mg/kg, i.e. 180 mg. Such a wide range illustrates the point made in the introduction that children cannot be regarded as 'scaled-down' adults when considering dosage and that more precise methods must be used for drugs with a narrow therapeutic range.

PAEDIATRIC DOSES CALCULATED BY BODY WEIGHT

The use of body weight is a better way of calculating doses for children than using the percentage methods discussed above. This is because it more accurately reflects the development of the child. Therefore, many children's doses are expressed as mg/kg. The method is not without its problems, particularly when dealing with obese children. In such situations, the dose prescribed would be greater than for a normal child of the same age. Therefore it is normally better to calculate the dose using the ideal body weight for the age, rather than the actual weight.

Example 12.2

A 7-year old child weighing 29 kg is prescribed chloroquine. Calculate the dose based on the actual weight and the ideal weight of the child.

The BNF indicates that for children of 4–7 years (body weight 16–25 kg) the dose is 150 mg weekly, and for children aged 8–12 years (body weight 25–45 kg) the dose is 225 mg weekly. Based on age, this child should receive 150 mg weekly, whilst based on weight the dose should be 225 mg. The lower dose is more reliable due to the obesity.

Example 12.3

The same child as in Example 12.2 is prescribed prochlorperazine, 250 micrograms/kg twice daily. What dose should the pharmacist recommend?

The child weighs 29 kg, therefore the dose = 29 × 0.250 mg = 7.25 mg. However, a child of 7 years should weigh 23 kg. When this figure is used to calculate the dose, a lower figure is obtained; dose = 23 × 0.250 mg = 5.75 mg. The lower dose is safer to recommend to the prescriber.

PAEDIATRIC DOSES USING BODY SURFACE AREA

It is recognized that the use of body surface area is the most accurate basis for calculating the dose of a drug for a child. The BNF uses body surface area as the basis for indicating normal children's doses for relatively few drugs, mostly chemotherapeutic agents, which have a very narrow therapeutic range. However, the surface area is not as easily determined as the weight of a child, so it presents a greater problem in calculating a suitable dose. The BNF gives values for anticipated body surface area in relation to age and height (Table 12.1). In addition, there are two other methods commonly used to calculate body surface area.

Calculation from weight and height

The body surface area can be calculated from body weight and height using the equation given below:

$$\text{Body surface area (m}^2) = \text{Weight (kg)}^{0.425} + \text{Height (cm)}^{0.725} \times 0.007184$$

Because the equation is cumbersome to use, the nomogram method is more commonly used.

Calculation of dose using a nomogram

The nomogram is shown in Figure 12.1. It is derived using the above equation, but is expressed as a nomogram to enable the body surface area to be read quickly when height and weight are known. To use the nomogram a ruler, or other straight edge, is lined up between the weight of the child (right hand scale) and the height of the child (left hand scale). The body surface area is read at the point on the central scale at which the ruler crosses it.

Example 12.4
A child has a height of 65 cm and a weight of 7.2 kg. What is the body surface area of the child?

Align the ruler between the two values on the nomogram. It intersects the surface area line at a value of 0.37 m^2. This is the body surface area of the child.

Example 12.5
A child of weight 9.4 kg and height 72 cm is prescribed 45 mg/m^2 tretinoin in two divided doses. What dose of drug should be given? Tretinoin is available in 10 mg capsules. What dosage regimen should be recommended?

Using the nomogram in Figure 12.1, we find that the body surface area of this child is 0.44 m^2. Therefore the daily dose required is $0.44 \times 45 = 19.8$ mg. This is to be given in two divided doses, that is:

$$\frac{19.8}{2} = 9.9 \text{ mg per dose.}$$

A 10 mg capsule is available, so one capsule should be taken twice a day. The BNF indicates warning label 21, indicating that each dose should be taken with or after food.

Example 12.6
A child is prescribed one 10 mg tablet of methotrexate to be taken each week. On checking the notes, you find that the child is two and a half years old, is 2 feet 9 inches tall and weighs 12 kg. Comment on the suitability of the dose. (The BNF oral dose for methotrexate for children with leukaemia is 15 mg/m^2 weekly.)

First, convert the child's height into centimetres (1 inch = 2.54 cm). 2 feet 9 inches = 33 inches, therefore 33×2.54 cm = 83.8 cm. Using the nomogram, we find that the body surface area is 0.53 m^2. From the BNF the dose of methotrexate is 15 mg/m^2, therefore the recommended dose is $15 \times 0.53 = 7.95$ mg.

The prescribed dose of 10 mg is high, and so should be queried with the prescriber.

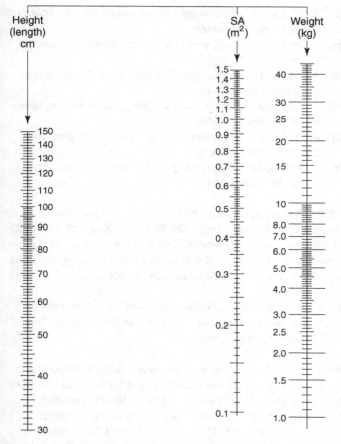

Height
(length)
cm

SA
(m²)

Weight
(kg)

Fig. 12.1 Nomogram relating weight, height and body surface area (SA) of children. (From *A Paediatric Vade-Mecum*, 13th edition, Arnold, 1996)

SELF-STUDY QUESTIONS

12.1 Using appropriate equations for calculating a child's dose as a proportion of the adult dose, calculate the dose for:

(a) A child age 7 years, weight 25 kg, height 121 cm, when the adult dose is 100 mg

(b) A child age 3 years, weight 15 kg, height 90 cm, when the adult dose is 50 mg

(c) A child age 6 years, weight 50 lb, height 44 in, when the adult dose is 75 mg

(d) A child age 1 year, weight 10.5 kg, height 75 cm, when the adult dose is 10 mg

(e) A child age 6 months, weight 7.8 kg, height 66 cm, when the adult dose is 500 mg

(f) A child age 8 years, weight 26 kg, height 129 cm, when the adult dose is 200 mg

(g) A child age 9 months, weight 9 kg, height 72 cm, when the adult dose is 40 mg

12.2 A child age 3 years and weighing 17 kg is prescribed chloroquine 62.5 mg weekly. The BNF indicates that for a child of 1–3 years and body weight 10–16 kg the dose is 112.5 mg weekly and age 4–7 years with body weight 16–25 kg the dose is 150 mg weekly. Provide advice on the dosage.

12.3 Ketoconazole is being prescribed for a 6-month-old infant who weighs 8 kg. What dose is recommended? (The BNF indicates 3 mg/kg daily.)

12.4 A child of 6 years is to be given oseltamivir. Compare the dose derived from ideal body weight for age and that from actual weight (the child weighs 31 pounds) with the BNF recommendations of under 15 kg: 30 mg every 12 hours; 16–23 kg: 45 mg every 12 hours; 24–40 kg: 60 mg every 12 hours.

12.5 A child age 1 year and weighing 11 kg is prescribed proguanil hydrochloride 75 mg daily. The BNF indicates that for an infant of 12 weeks to 11 months and body weight 6–10 kg the dose is 50 mg daily, and age 1–3 years with body weight 10–16 kg the dose is 75 mg daily. Give advice on the dosage.

12.6 An epileptic child of 7 years, weighing 19 kg, is to be given diazepam. The BNF suggests a dose of

200–300 µg/kg or 1 mg per year of age. What dose should be recommended?

12.7 A child with epilepsy is to be prescribed phenytoin 5 mg/kg in 2 divided doses. The child is 4 years old and weighs 17 kg. What dose is required?

12.8 An autistic child is being prescribed chlorpromazine hydrochloride 500 µ/kg every 4–6 hours to a maximum of 40 mg daily for a child aged 1–5. The child is 3 feet tall, weighs 2 stones 6 pounds and is of normal build. What dose is required?

12.9 Calculate the dose of drug for each child detailed:

(a) Zidovudine to provide 120 mg/m^2 for a patient of estimated surface area 0.32 m^2
(b) Cisplatin to provide 60 mg/m^2 for a patient of estimated surface area 0.66 m^2
(c) Daunorubicin to provide 25 mg/m^2 for a patient of estimated surface area 0.75 m^2
(d) Somatropin to provide 21 units/m^2 for a patient of estimated surface area 0.54 m^2

12.10 A baby weighing 5 kg requires 7.5 mg/kg clarithromycin twice daily for 7 days. A paediatric suspension containing 125 mg/5 mL is available. What dose is required? How much suspension should be dispensed?

12.11 A child weighing 12 kg is prescribed 62.5 mg/kg terbinafine once daily for 3 weeks. Tablets containing 250 mg are commercially available. Calculate the individual dose, dose regimen and number of tablets required.

12.12 A neonate weighing 3.2 kg requires an infusion containing benzylpenicillin, 50 mg/kg, twice daily. How much benzylpenicillin will be administered by each infusion?

12.13 Along with other drugs, a child of height 121 cm and weight 9.6 kg is to be given ritonavir 250 mg/m^2 every

12 hours, increased by 50 mg/m^2 every 3 days to 350 mg/m^2 which will be maintained for 2 weeks. 100 mg capsules and an oral solution containing 400 mg/5 mL are available. Calculate the dosage regimen and the number or volume of medicine required (using an oral syringe calibrated in 0.1 mL graduations if required).

12.14   In combination with other antiretroviral drugs a 9-year-old child is being prescribed nevirapine at a dose of 4 mg/kg daily for 14 days then 4 mg/kg twice daily for 14 days. A suspension containing 50 mg/5 mL is available. What doses are required and how much medicine should be supplied?

12.15   Following renal transplantation a 12-year-old child is to receive 600 mg/m^2 mycophenolate mofetil twice daily for 2 weeks. The BNF indicates '2–18 years (and body surface area over 1.25 m^2) 600 mg/m^2 twice daily (maximum 2 g daily)'. The following dosage forms are available: capsules 250 mg, tablets 500 mg, oral suspension 1 g/5 mL. Calculate the dose and the amount of a suitable dosage form to supply.

12.16   An infant, aged 9 months, is to receive didanosine at a rate of 240 mg/m^2 in 2 divided doses for 3 weeks. The child is 27 inches tall and weighs 18 pounds. What dose is required? The BNF indicates that only Videx tablets (available at 25 mg and 200 mg strength) can be used for an infant of this age. What dosage regimen should be used and how many tablets should be supplied?

For answers to these questions see page 288

Reconstitution for oral and parenteral use

After studying this chapter you will be able to:
- Calculate the concentration produced by reconstituting oral and injection preparations
- Calculate the volumes required to provide specific doses
- Take account of the displacement volume of the drug when reconstituting injections
- Allow for the volume occupied by other ingredients in oral medicines

INTRODUCTION

Some drugs are not chemically stable in solution and so are supplied as dry powders for reconstitution just before use. Many of these are antibiotics, but there is also a range of chemotherapeutic agents used in cancer treatment. The antibiotics may be for oral use or for injection. An oral antibiotic for reconstitution comes as a powder in a bottle with sufficient space to add the water. The powder itself will remain stable for up to two years when dry. When reconstituted, a shelf life of 10–14 days is normal, depending on whether it is kept in the refrigerator or not. If larger volumes are added to reduce the final concentration, this may affect the efficacy of any preservatives. Drugs for injection are equally stable when dry, but are to be used within hours of reconstitution. Because they are for injection they are sterile powders and are dissolved in sterile water aseptically. There are a number of calculations which may be required around the reconstitution processes.

Example 13.1

What dose of antibiotic will be contained in a 5 mL spoonful when a bottle containing 5 g of penicillin V is reconstituted to give 200 mL of syrup?

For this type of calculation, the simple proportion equation can be used;

$$\frac{Wt_1}{Wt_2} = \frac{Vol_1}{Vol_2}$$

5 g = 5000 mg

Let y be the weight (in mg) in 5 mL. Substituting:

$$\frac{5000 \text{ mg}}{y \text{ mg}} = \frac{200 \text{ mL}}{5 \text{ mL}}, \text{ therefore } y = \frac{5000 \times 5}{200} = 125 \text{ mg}$$

Sometimes, the doctor may request a more or less concentrated syrup to be produced which requires altering the amount of water added from that indicated by the manufacturer.

Example 13.2

An ampicillin product is available for reconstitution. It contains 2.5 g of ampicillin to be made up to 100 mL. To what volume should it be made to give 100 mg per 5 mL dose?

Let y be the weight (in mg) in 5 mL of the normal mixture. The normal mixture will give a dose of:

$$\frac{2500 \text{ mg}}{y \text{ mg}} = \frac{100 \text{ mL}}{5 \text{ mL}}$$

$$\text{Therefore } y = \frac{2500 \times 5}{100} = 125 \text{ mg per 5 mL}$$

To calculate the final volume (z), the same equation is used:

$$\frac{2500 \text{ mg}}{100 \text{ mg}} = \frac{z \text{ mL}}{5 \text{ mL}}, \text{ therefore } z = \frac{2500 \times 5}{100} = 125 \text{ mL}$$

This type of oral mixture is likely to have other ingredients—thickeners, colours, flavours, etc., as well as the actual drug, all of which will occupy some of the final volume. So it is necessary to be able to calculate exactly how much water to add.

Example 13.3

The label on an ampicillin bottle indicates that 78 mL of water must be added to produce 100 mL of final syrup. How much water must be added to give the 125 mL final volume?

Thus, the volume of powder in the final syrup:
100 mL – 78 mL = 22 mL. Therefore, the volume to add to give 125 mL is 125 mL – 22 mL = 103 mL.

Example 13.4

A child weighing 60 lb requires a dose of 8 mg/kg of ampicillin. Given that a 5 mL dose is to be given, what volume of water must be added when the powder is reconstituted?

Instructions on the label indicate that dilution to 150 mL (by adding 111 mL) gives 250 mg ampicillin per 5 mL.

Conversion of weight to kg: 60/2.2 = 27.27 kg.
Calculation of amount of ampicillin required: $27.27 \times 8 = 218$ mg.
Calculation of amount of ampicillin in container (y):

$$\frac{250 \text{ mg}}{y \text{ mg}} = \frac{5 \text{ mL}}{150 \text{ mL}}, \text{ therefore } y = \frac{250 \times 150}{5} = 7500 \text{ mg} = 7.5 \text{ g}.$$

Calculation of final volume (z) to give 218 mg per 5 mL:

$$\frac{218 \text{ mg}}{7500 \text{ mg}} = \frac{5 \text{ mL}}{z \text{ mL}}, \text{ therefore } z = \frac{7500 \times 5}{218} = 172 \text{ mL}.$$

Volume occupied by powder is 150 mL – 111 mL = 39 mL. Therefore the volume to be added is 172 mL – 39 mL = 133 mL.

DISPLACEMENT VOLUME

Drugs for injection solutions do not normally contain ingredients other than the drug (or they make an insignificant contribution to the final volume). However, there is another problem which has to be recognized because it is more significant with the more potent drugs used for injections. When any drug is dissolved, it takes up a finite volume in the final solution. In many cases this is such a small volume that it is of no significance. However, if the volume of solvent displaced is significant, then this volume must be allowed for. This is especially important when the final volume produced is relatively small, because it represents a larger percentage of the total volume. When reconstituting injections, water for injections must be added aseptically to produce the required final volume, i.e. water for injections cannot be added 'to' a final volume. Thus, it has to be possible to calculate exactly how much water for injections is to be measured in a syringe for adding. The final volume of solution may not be specified by the manufacturer and is a matter for decision by the pharmacist depending on the way the resulting injection is to be used.

To make the appropriate calculations, it is necessary to know the volume of water for injections which will be displaced by a known weight of the drug. This is called the displacement volume. *The Pharmaceutical Codex* (12th edition) has a table listing the displacement values. Alternatively, manufacturers' product information will include the information.

Example 13.5

A vial containing 100 mg hydrocortisone sodium succinate powder for injection is to be reconstituted to produce 2 mL of injection. How much water for injections should be added to the powder? The displacement volume of hydrocortisone sodium succinate is given in *The Pharmaceutical Codex* as 0.05 mL/100 mg.

The displacement volume indicates that 100 mg of hydrocortisone sodium succinate will occupy the volume of 0.05 mL of water for injections in the final solution. Therefore, the volume of water for injections to be added is 2.00 − 0.05 = 1.95 mL.

Example 13.6

Cyclophosphamide is available in vials containing 200 mg, 500 mg or 1 g. Given that the displacement volume is 0.1 mL/100 mg, calculate the volume of water for injections to be added to produce 25 mL injections from each of the vials.

The displacement volume given for cyclophosphamide is for 100 mg, but the vials contain larger quantities. The displacement volume for the larger weights can be calculated by simple proportion.
Let the volume displaced by the 200 mg, 500 mg and 1 g be x, y and z respectively.

For 200 mg injection:

$$\frac{100}{0.1} = \frac{200}{x}, \text{ therefore } x = \frac{200 \times 0.1}{100} = 0.2 \text{ mL.}$$

Therefore the volume of water for injections is 25 − 0.2 = 24.8 mL.

For 500 mg injection:

$$\frac{100}{0.1} = \frac{500}{y}, \text{ therefore } y = \frac{500 \times 0.1}{100} = 0.5 \text{ mL.}$$

Therefore the volume of water for injections is 25 − 0.5 = 24.5 mL.

For 1 g injection, convert drug weight to milligrams:

$$\frac{100}{0.1} = \frac{1000}{z}, \text{ therefore } z = \frac{1000 \times 0.1}{100} = 1.0 \text{ mL.}$$

Therefore the volume of water for injections is 25 − 1.0 = 24.0 mL.

Example 13.7

A patient requires an injection of 50 mg doxorubicin containing 2.5 mg/mL. What volume of water for injections should be added to the 50 mg vial? The displacement volume is 0.03 mL/10 mg.

The first part of this question is to work out the final volume of the injection. This is done by using simple proportion. Let the volume of final injection be y. Therefore

$$\frac{2.5}{1} = \frac{50}{y}, \; y = \frac{50 \times 1}{2.5} = 20 \text{ mL.}$$

The second part of the question requires the calculation of the volume of water for injections which will be displaced by 50 mg of doxorubicin. Let the volume displaced be z. Therefore

$$\frac{0.03}{10} = \frac{z}{50}, \; z = \frac{0.03 \times 50}{10} = 0.15 \text{ mL.}$$

Finally, the volume of water for injections to be added to the 50 mg doxorubicin can be calculated: 20 − 0.15 = 19.85 mL.

SELF-STUDY QUESTIONS

13.1 What is the weight of antibiotic in a 5 mL dose when a bottle containing the stated weight of antibiotic is reconstituted as indicated?

(a) 5 g antibiotic is made up with water to give 50 mL of syrup
(b) 15 g antibiotic is made up with water to give 150 mL of syrup
(c) 5 g antibiotic is made up with water to give 200 mL of syrup
(d) 20 g antibiotic is made up with water to give 160 mL of syrup

(e) 15 g antibiotic is made up with water to give 200 mL of syrup

13.2 What is the weight of antibiotic in a 15 mL dose when a bottle containing the stated weight of antibiotic is reconstituted as indicated?

(a) 15 g antibiotic is made up with water to give 75 mL of syrup
(b) 5 g antibiotic is made up with water to give 125 mL of syrup
(c) 20 g antibiotic is made up with water to give 300 mL of syrup

13.3 What is the total volume, after adding water to the stated weight of antibiotic, to provide the required amount per 5 mL dose?

(a) 2.5 g of antibiotic to give 100 mg dose
(b) 15 g of antibiotic to give 250 mg dose
(c) 10 g of antibiotic to give 400 mg dose
(d) 25 g of antibiotic to give 500 mg dose

13.4 What is the total volume, after adding water to the stated weight of antibiotic, to provide the required amount per 15 mL dose?

(a) 12 g of antibiotic to give 800 mg dose
(b) 2.5 g of antibiotic to give 375 mg dose
(c) 18 g of antibiotic to give 300 mg dose

13.5 A bottle is reconstituted as shown. What dose is contained in 5 mL?

(a) 10 g of antibiotic made up to 100 mL
(b) 5 g of antibiotic made up to 200 mL
(c) 20 g of antibiotic made up to 400 mL

13.6 A bottle is reconstituted as shown. What dose is contained in 10 mL?

(a) 25 g of antibiotic is made up to 200 mL
(b) 12 g of antibiotic is made up to 150 mL

(c) 20 g of antibiotic is made up to 500 mL

13.7 The label on a bottle of an antibiotic for reconstitution indicates the volume of water to be added to make 100 mL of syrup. How much water should be added to produce the specified volume?

(a) 78 mL on label, 110 mL of syrup required
(b) 87 mL on label, 120 mL of syrup required
(c) 92 mL on label, 130 mL of syrup required
(d) 78 mL on label, 170 mL of syrup required
(e) 87 mL on label, 140 mL of syrup required
(f) 92 mL on label, 90 mL of syrup required
(g) 89 mL on label, 115 mL of syrup required

13.8 An injection is to be added to a sterile solution to produce a 500 mL infusion. Calculate the amount to be added:

(a) Amphotericin containing 50 mg/10 mL to produce a 1 mg/mL infusion
(b) Amphotericin containing 50 mg/10 mL to produce a 1200 µg/mL infusion
(c) Amphotericin containing 50 mg/10 mL to produce a 200 µg/mL infusion
(d) Colomycin containing 500 000 units/mL to produce an infusion containing 105 000 units/mL
(e) Colomycin containing 1000 000 units/mL to produce an infusion containing 150 000 units/mL.

13.9 The label on a bottle of an antibiotic syrup indicates the volume of water that should be added to produce a given strength of reconstituted syrup. Calculate the total amount of water to be added to produce the syrup of different strength.

(a) 92 mL of water gives 100 mL of syrup containing 125 mg/5 mL. A syrup of 100 mg/5 mL is required.
(b) 87 mL of water gives 100 mL of syrup containing 250 mg/5 mL. A syrup of 200 mg/5 mL is required.
(c) 128 mL of water gives 140 mL of syrup containing 125 mg/5 mL. A syrup of 100 mg/5 mL is required.

(d) 89 mL of water gives 100 mL of syrup containing 500 mg/5 mL. A syrup of 400 mg/5 mL is required.

(e) 87 mL of water gives 100 mL of syrup containing 200 mg/5 mL. A syrup of 250 mg/5 mL is required.

13.10 How much water is required to reconstitute the following injections?

(a) A vial contains 500 mg ampicillin for reconstitution to produce 5 mL. (The displacement volume of ampicillin is 0.2 mL/250 mg.)

(b) A vial contains 1.2 g co-amoxiclav for reconstitution to produce 20 mL. (The displacement volume of co-amoxiclav is 0.5 mL/600 mg.)

(c) A vial contains 1 g chloramphenicol for reconstitution to produce 40 mL. (The displacement volume of chloramphenicol is 0.8 mL.)

13.11 Some injections for reconstitution are available in different sizes. For each of the following, calculate the volume of water for injections to be added:

(a) 5 mg, 30 mg and 100 mg of diamorphine to be made to 20 mL. (The displacement volume of diamorphine is 0.06 mL/5 mg.)

(b) 300 mg and 600 mg of rifampicin to be made to a volume of 10 mL. (The displacement volume of rifampicin is 0.24 mL/300 mg.)

(c) 1 g and 5 g of treosulfan to be made to a volume of 100 mL. (The displacement volume of treosulfan is 2.5 mL/5 g.)

(d) 2.25 g, and 4.5 g of tazocin to be made to a volume of 30 mL. (The displacement volume of tazocin is 0.7 mL/g.)

13.12 Glucagon, 1 mg, is available with a pre-filled syringe for reconstitution to 1 mL. The displacement volume is 0.04 mL/mg. What volume of water for injections is in the syringe?

13.13 A vial for reconstitution contains the stated weight. What volume of water is required to produce the injection?

(a) 400 mg of sodium valproate is to be reconstituted to produce a solution of 100 mg/mL. (The displacement volume of sodium valproate is 0.35 mL/400 mg.)

(b) 50 mg of azathioprine is to be reconstituted to produce a solution of 10 mg/mL. (The displacement volume of azathioprine is 0.05 mL/50 mg.)

(c) 20 mg of hydralazine is to be reconstituted to produce 1 mL of a 2% solution. (The displacement volume of hydralazine is 0.14 mL/20 mg.)

For answers to these questions see page 290

CHAPTER

14

Calculations associated with injections

After studying this chapter you will be able to:

- **Complete the calculations for making solutions isotonic with body fluids using the freezing point depression method**
- **Calculate the quantities of drug solutions to use as intravenous additives**
- **Determine required infusion rates and express these as millilitres per minute or drops per minute**
- **Calculate the time it will take to administer an infusion of known volume**
- **Understand the principles in compounding total parenteral infusion fluids**

This chapter will deal with two main groups of calculations: those involved in making a solution isotonic and those used in preparing and administering intravenous infusions.

ISOTONIC SOLUTIONS

When a solute is dissolved in a solvent, the presence of the solute alters the colligative properties of the solvent. Thus there is a lowering of vapour pressure, elevation of boiling point, depression of freezing point and increase of osmotic pressure. All these depend on the total number of particles in solution, irrespective of whether they are ions, molecules or both. The most important of these properties is the osmotic pressure because it relates to fluid transport across physiological membranes. When two solutions have the same osmotic pressure they are said to be iso-osmotic or isotonic. In pharmacy, isotonic solutions have the same osmotic

181

pressure as blood plasma and do not damage the membrane of red blood cells. Hypotonic solutions have a lower osmotic pressure than blood plasma and cause blood cells to swell and burst because of fluids passing into the cells by osmosis. Hypertonic solutions have a higher osmotic pressure than plasma; as a result the red blood cells lose fluids and shrink. Following the administration of an injection it is important that tissue damage, irritation and haemolysis of red blood cells are minimized. Thus, the *British Pharmacopoeia* states that aqueous solutions for large-volume infusion fluids, together with aqueous fluids for subcutaneous, intradermal and intramuscular administration, should be made isotonic. Intrathecal injections must also be isotonic to avoid serious changes in the osmotic pressure of the cerebrospinal fluid.

Eye drops should also be made isotonic to avoid the sting associated with non-isotonic solutions applied to the eyes. Aqueous hypotonic solutions are made isotonic by adding either sodium chloride, glucose or, occasionally, mannitol. The latter two agents are incompatible with some drugs. If the solution is hypertonic it is made isotonic by dilution.

Making solutions isotonic

Injection solutions are often made isotonic with 0.9% w/v sodium chloride solution. The amount of solute, or the required dilution necessary to make a solution isotonic, can be determined by a number of different methods. The most common of these is the freezing point depression.

Freezing point depression

The freezing point depression of blood plasma and tears is 0.52°C. Thus solutions that freeze at –0.52°C have the same osmotic pressure as body fluids. Hypotonic solutions have a smaller freezing point depression and require the addition of a solute to depress the freezing point to –0.52°C.

The amount of adjusting substance to be added to these solutions may be calculated from the equation:

$$W = \frac{(0.52 - a)}{b}$$

where W = percentage concentration of adjusting substance in the final solution, that is g per 100 mL, a = freezing point depression of the unadjusted hypotonic solution (calculated by multiplying the depression of a 1% solution by the % concentration of the solution), b = freezing point depression of a 1% w/v concentration of the adjusting substance.

An extensive list of freezing point depression values is detailed in *The Pharmaceutical Codex* (1994) on pages 53–64.

Example 14.1

A 200 mL volume of a 2% w/v solution of glucose for intravenous injection is to be made isotonic by the addition of sodium chloride.

From *The Pharmaceutical Codex*, a 1% w/v solution of glucose (anhydrous) depresses the freezing point of water by 0.100°C and a 1% solution of sodium chloride depresses the freezing point of water by 0.576°C.

The depression of freezing point of the unadjusted solution of glucose (a in the equation) will therefore be:

$$a = 2 \times 0.100 = 0.2.$$

A 1% w/v solution of sodium chloride depresses the freezing point of water by 0.576°C (b in the equation). Substituting these values for a and b in the above equation:

$$W = \frac{(0.52 - 0.2)}{0.576} = \frac{0.32}{0.576} = 0.556 \text{ g per 100 mL.}$$

The intravenous solution thus requires the addition of 0.556 g of sodium chloride per 100 mL volume to make it isotonic with blood plasma. The request is for 200 mL. Therefore the amount of sodium chloride required = $0.556 \times 2 = 1.11$ g.

Other methods of calculating for isotonicity

Other methods that are used to estimate the amount of adjusting substances required to make a solution isotonic include:

- sodium chloride equivalents
- molar concentrations
- serum osmolarity.

Details of these methods are given in the chapter 'Solution properties' in the twelfth edition of *The Pharmaceutical Codex* (1994, pp. 64–67). Care is required when using different methods for calculating isotonicity because the units used by the different methods are not the same. For example, the freezing point depression method uses percentages and gives an answer in grams per 100 mL, whereas the sodium chloride equivalents method uses units of g per litre. It should also be noted that the methods are approximations, so slightly different answers will be given. It is true that using the differing quantities will produce solutions of slightly different tonicity, but these differences are of no clinical significance.

Example 14.2

Prepare 15 mL of isotonic 2% pilocarpine hydrochloride eye drops

From *The Pharmaceutical Codex*, a 1% solution of pilocarpine hydrochloride depresses the freezing point of water by 0.134°C. Therefore a 2% solution causes a depression of 2 × 0.134 = 0.268°C (*a* in the equation).

A 1% solution of sodium chloride depresses the freezing point of water by 0.576°C (*b* in the equation). Substituting:

$$W = \frac{(0.52 - 0.268)}{0.576} = \frac{0.252}{0.576} = 0.4375 \text{ g per 100 mL}$$

The request is for 15 mL of eye drops, therefore we require

$$\frac{0.4375 \times 15}{100} = 0.0656\,\text{g} = 0.066\,\text{g} = 66 \text{ mg}$$

Example 14.3

Calculate the quantities required to prepare an injection to the following formula:

Atropine sulphate	60 mg
Morphine sulphate	1 g
Sodium metabisulphite	100 mg
Water for injections	to 100 mL

The Pharmaceutical Codex gives the following depressions of freezing point for 1% solutions:

Atropine sulphate	0.073°C
Morphine sulphate	0.078°C
Sodium metabisulphite	0.389°C

The units for the weight of the ingredients must be the same, preferably grams because these are the units used in the equation.

Therefore atropine sulphate is 0.06 g and sodium metabisulphite is 0.1 g.

To obtain a figure for 'a' in the equation, the depression caused by each of the ingredients must be calculated and added together.

Atropine sulphate depression = $0.06 \times 0.073 = 0.00438°C$

Morphine sulphate depression = $1 \times 0.078 = 0.078°C$

Sodium metabisulphite depression = $0.1 \times 0.389 = 0.0389°C$

Therefore the total depression of freezing point from the three ingredients is:

$0.00438 + 0.078 + 0.0389 = 0.12128°C$ (this is a in the equation)

Substituting:

$$W = \frac{(0.52 - 0.12128)}{0.576} = \frac{0.39872}{0.576} = 0.692 \text{ g per 100 mL.}$$

Therefore 0.692 g of sodium chloride must be added to the formula when making the 100 mL injection solution.

INTRAVENOUS ADDITIVES

Chapter 13 considered the reconstitution of drugs which are produced by the manufacturer as a dry powder for reconstitution shortly before use. These drugs are frequently then given to patients intravenously by adding them to an intravenous infusion fluid. Some drugs will have a significant displacement volume, which would have to be allowed for when reconstituting the solution. Subsequent calculations include working out how much drug solution should be added to an infusion fluid, what concentration, in mg/mL, is produced, then working out the speed of infusion, in terms of either mg/min or mL/min and how this is achieved when it is being administered by means of a giving set.

Example 14.4

An ampoule of flucloxacillin contains 250 mg of powder with instructions to produce a 5 mL solution with water for injections. What volume of this solution should be added to 500 mL of saline infusion to provide a dose of 175 mg? What is the concentration, in mg/mL, produced?

250 mg in 5 mL = 50 mg per mL. Therefore, volume for 175 mg:

$$\frac{175}{50} = 3.5 \text{ mL}.$$

In preparing the infusion, 3.5 mL is added to 500 mL of normal saline infusion. This produces a total volume of 503.5 mL. Therefore there is 175 mg in 503.5 mL (not 500 mL). Division obtains the concentration of the resulting infusion:

$$\text{Concentration of flucloxacillin} = \frac{175}{503.5} = 0.348 = 0.35 \text{ mg/mL}$$

Note: Whenever a solution is added to a pre-prepared infusion, the volumes of the two solutions must be added together to give the total volume of the resulting infusion.

Example 14.5

A patient with deep-vein thrombosis is to receive an infusion of streptokinase. A vial containing 1.5 million units of streptokinase powder is available. It should be dissolved in sterile saline to produce 50 mL. Sufficient amount of this solution is to be added to 500 mL saline infusion to produce a concentration of 2000 units per mL. How much of the reconstituted solution should be added to the saline infusion?

The difficulty with this calculation is that, as the streptokinase concentrate is added to the saline infusion it increases the volume and so more of the concentrate is required to produce the target concentration. This is the same sort of problem which was dealt with in Chapter 8 using alligation. The same method can be used in this example.

As the question is stated, two different methods of expressing concentration are used: the concentrate is 1.5 million units per 50 mL and the required solution is 2000 units per mL. Before using alligation, the units must be made the same.

Convert the concentration of the reconstituted streptokinase to units/mL:

$$\text{Concentration} = \frac{1500\ 000}{50} = 30\ 000 \text{ units/mL}.$$

It is now possible to carry out the alligation, using the concentrate and saline (0% streptokinase) as starting solutions and 2000 units/mL as the target solution:

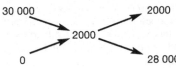

Thus we require 2000 parts of the concentrate and 28 000 parts of the normal saline infusion. However, we know that the volume of the infusion is 500 mL, therefore 28 000 parts equals 500 mL. Next calculate the volume of 1 part:

$$= \frac{500}{28\,000} = 0.017857 \text{ mL}.$$

2000 parts of concentrate are required, therefore $2000 \times 0.017857 = 35.71$ mL. Thus 35.71 mL of reconstituted streptokinase is added to 500 mL of normal saline to produce an infusion of total volume 535.71 mL.

Note: This answer can be checked by working backwards as illustrated in Chapter 8:

35.71 mL of concentrate contains $\dfrac{1500\,000 \times 35.71}{50} = 1071\,300$ units of streptokinase.

These 1071 300 units are dissolved in 535.71 mL, therefore the concentration produced is

$$\frac{1071\,300}{535.71} = 2000 \text{ units per mL}.$$

Example 14.6

Calculate the number of millimoles of magnesium and chloride ions in 1 litre of a 2% magnesium chloride (hexahydrate) infusion fluid.

1 litre of 2% solution contains 20 g of magnesium chloride. Magnesium chloride is $MgCl_2.6H_2O$ with a molecular weight of 203.3. Using the equation given in Chapter 2:

$$\% \text{ w/v} = (W \times M)/10\,000$$

where W is the number of milligrams of salt containing 1 mmol of the required ion and M is the number of millimoles per litre. Substituting:

$$2 = \frac{203.3 \times M}{10\,000}, \text{ therefore } M = \frac{2 \times 10\,000}{203.3} = 98.38 \text{ mmol}.$$

Each mole of magnesium chloride provides 1 mole of magnesium ions and 2 moles of chloride ions. Thus, 1 litre of the solution contains 98.4 mmol of magnesium ions and 196.8 mmol of chloride ions.

Example 14.7

Calculate the number of millimoles of dextrose and sodium ions in 1 litre of sodium chloride and dextrose injection containing 5% w/v anhydrous dextrose and 0.9% w/v of sodium chloride

Use the conversion equation for % w/v calculations (see Ch. 2 and Example 14.6):

$$\% \ w/v = (W \times M)/10\ 000$$

Rearranging this equation:

$$M = \% \ w/v \times 10\ 000/W$$

For dextrose:

$$W = 180.2, \text{ therefore } M = \frac{5.0 \times 10\ 000}{180.2} = 277 \text{ mmol}$$

Thus 1 litre of solution contains 277 mmol of dextrose.
For sodium chloride:

$$M = \frac{0.9 \times 10\ 000}{58.44} = 154 \text{ mmol}$$

As 1 mmol of sodium chloride provides 1 mmol of both sodium and chloride ions, 1 litre of the solution will contain 154 mmol of both sodium and chloride ions.

Example 14.8
Calculate the quantities of salts required for the following electrolyte solution:

Sodium	12 mmol
Potassium	4 mmol
Magnesium	6 mmol
Calcium	6 mmol
Chloride	40 mmol

Water for injections to 1 L
From Table 4 in *The Pharmaceutical Codex* (12th edition, p. 49):

- 12 mmol of sodium ions are provided by 12×58.44 mg of sodium chloride that also yields 12 mmol of chloride.
- 4 mmol of potassium ions are provided by 4×74.55 mg of potassium chloride, which also yields 4 mmol of chloride ions.
- 6 mmol of magnesium ions are provided by 6×203.3 mg of magnesium chloride, which also yields $2 \times 6 = 12$ mmol of chloride ions as there are two chloride ions in the molecule.
- 6 mmol of calcium ions are provided by 6×147.0 mg of calcium chloride (dihydrate), which also yields 12 mmol of chloride ions as there are two chloride ions in the molecule.
- 40 mmol of chloride ions are obtained from the individual salts (sodium chloride, potassium chloride, magnesium chloride and calcium chloride respectively):

$$12 + 4 + 12 + 12 = 40 \text{ mmol of chloride ion}$$

The formula can, therefore, be shown as in Table 14.1. It should be noted that the charges on the anions and cations are equally balanced.

Table 14.1 The formula for Example 14.8

	Weight	Na$^+$	K$^+$	Mg^{2+}	Ca^{2+}	Cl$^-$
		Millimoles of:				
Sodium chloride	$12 \times 58.44 = 701$ mg	12				12
Potassium chloride	$4 \times 74.55 = 298$ mg		4			4
Magnesium chloride	$6 \times 203.3 = 1220$ mg			6		12
Calcium chloride	$6 \times 147.0 = 882$ mg				6	12
Water for injections	to 1 L					
Total (mmol/L)		12	4	6	6	40

RATE OF INFUSION

When administering intravenous infusions, the rate of addition is first calculated in terms of millilitres per minute. Once this figure has been calculated, the duration of infusion can be calculated in the form required and the rate can be either used directly, or converted into appropriate information for the nurse setting up the infusion.

Infusions are administered using either a pump driver or a giving set with a drip chamber in the tube. There are different designs of pump drivers, but they all permit the setting of a rate of infusion in terms of millilitres per minute or millilitres per hour. With giving sets, administration uses gravity as the driving force. Partial clamping of the tube using a roller clamp allows the rate of dripping to be controlled. The drop size, that is drop volume, varies and is a property of the dimensions of the tip within the drip chamber. As the drop volume changes, so does the number of drops per millilitre. Standard giving sets at present have drop volumes of either 20 drops per millilitre or 60 drops per millilitre, although other drop volumes are possible. When the drop volume is known, the rate of millilitres per minute can be converted into drops per minute. The nurse can then adjust the giving set to the required rate of infusion.

Alternatively the doctor may specify the duration of the infusion, which will require the calculation of the rate of infusion and the infusion volume.

Example 14.9

An infusion contains 10 mL of a 1 in 5000 solution of isoprenaline hydrochloride and 500 mL of 5% dextrose solution. At what flow rate should this be given to provide 5 µg drug per minute and how long will the total infusion take?

10 ml of a 1 in 5000 solution contains 2 mg of isoprenaline hydrochloride. 2 mg = 2000 µg of drug in 500 + 10 = 510 mL of solution. Using simple proportion: let the number of millilitres containing 5 µg (to be administered in 1 min) be y. Then:

$$\frac{2000}{5} = \frac{510}{y} \text{, therefore } y = \frac{510 \times 5}{2000} = 1.275 \text{ ml/min}$$

The time required is also calculated by simple proportion. Let the time for the infusion be z, then:

$$\frac{1.275}{510} = \frac{1}{z} \text{, therefore } z = \frac{1 \times 510}{1.275} = 400 \text{ min.}$$

This can be converted into hours by dividing by 60: 400/60 = 6 hours 40 minutes.

Example 14.10

100 mg of metaraminol tartrate are added to 500 mL of saline infusion. What should be the rate of infusion to give a dose of 2 mg per minute? How long will the infusion take?

Using simple proportion:

$$\frac{100}{2} = \frac{500}{y} \text{, therefore } y = \frac{500 \times 2}{100} = 10 \text{ mL}$$

Therefore 10 mL contains the required amount of metaraminol tartrate. The infusion rate should be 10 mL per minute. The total volume is 500 mL, therefore the time taken at 10 mL/min is:

$$\frac{500}{10} = 50 \text{ min.}$$

Example 14.11

A patient was given an initial dose of mexiletine hydrochloride following myocardial infarction. He is now to be initiated on an infusion using the standard 0.1% solution at a rate of 250 mg for the first hour, then 125 mg per hour for 2 hours and then 500 micrograms per minute. What rates of infusion are required?

A 0.1% solution is 100 mg in 100 mL, that is 1 mg in 1 mL.

During the first hour the patient will require 250 mg, that is 250 mL of infusion. This infusion rate may be quoted as 250 mL/h or converted to mL/min by dividing by 60, giving a rate of 4.17 mL/min.

During the following two hours, the patient will receive 125 mL/h, or 2.08 mL/min.

Subsequently a rate giving 500 micrograms per minute is required. This is equivalent to $500 \times 60 = 30\,000$ micrograms per hour. This can be converted to milligrams by dividing by 1000, that is 30 mg/h. Therefore the patient will require 30 mL of infusion per hour, or 0.5 mL/min.

Example 14.12

A doctor requires an infusion of 1000 mL of 5% dextrose to be administered over an 8-hour period. Using an IV giving set which delivers 10 drops/mL, how many drops per minute should be delivered to the patient?

First convert the time into minutes:

$$8 \text{ hour} = 8 \times 60 \text{ min} = 480 \text{ min}$$

Next calculate how many mL/min are required:

$$\frac{1000}{480} = 2.08 \text{ mL/min.}$$

Then calculate the number of drops this requires:

$$2.08 \text{ mL/min} \times 10 \text{ drops/min} = 21 \text{ drops/min}$$

Example 14.13

A patient is to receive 5% dextrose by infusion using a giving set delivering 55 mL per hour. How much fluid will the patient receive over 2 hours, 3 hours and 6 hours?

A simple multiplication is required to provide the answers:

After 2 hours, the patient will have received $2 \times 55 = 110$ mL.
After 3 hours, the patient will have received $3 \times 55 = 165$ mL.
After 6 hours, the patient will have received $6 \times 55 = 330$ mL.

Example 14.14

A patient is to receive an infusion of 500 mL of Ringer's Solution. The infusion pump is set at 40 mL/h. How long will the infusion last?

The time taken is the volume divided by the rate, therefore

$$\frac{500}{40} = 12.5 \text{ hours}$$

This information is required so that the nurse knows when to either stop the infusion or change the bag if it is to continue for a longer duration.

Example 14.15

A 500 mL dextrose infusion is to be administered over 4 hours. The giving set available delivers 20 drops per millilitre. How many drops per minute should be administered?

First, convert the time into minutes and calculate the infusion rate:

$$Rate = \frac{500}{4 \times 60} = 2.08 \text{ mL/min}$$

Each millilitre will require 20 drops, therefore the drop rate is $2.08 \times 20 = 41.6$ drops per minute. The adjustable clamp should be set so that there are 42 drops per minute in the drip chamber.

Example 14.16

At 10 a.m. a 1 L bag of normal saline infusion is set up to be administered using an infusion pump at 70 mL/h. After 9 hours, the doctor requests that the flow rate be increased to 90 mL/h. At what time will the bag require replacing?

During the first 9 hours, $70 \times 9 = 630$ mL of saline infusion has been administered. Therefore, the amount of infusion remaining is $(1000 - 630) = 370$ mL. This volume is now to be administered at a rate of 90 mL/h. This will take $\frac{370}{90} = 4.11$ hours to administer— approximately 4 hours. The total infusion time for the 1 L bag is $(9 + 4) = 13$ hours. Since the injection started at 10 a.m., the bag will require replacement at 11 p.m.

Example 14.17

20 mL of a drug solution is added to a 500 mL infusion solution. It has to be administered to the patient over a 5-hour period using a set giving 15 drops per mL. How many drops per min are required?

This example is typical of those where a drug is being added to the infusion, whether reconstituted or manufactured as a solution. The calculation must take account of the increase in volume produced by the mixing of the two solutions.

First calculate the total volume of infusion:

$$20 + 500 = 520 \text{ mL}$$

Then calculate the number of drops which will be administered in total. This can be done because we know that each millilitre of infusion requires 15 drops:

Therefore, there will be 520×15 drops = 7800 drops

Next the duration of the infusion is expressed in minutes

$$5 \times 60 = 300 \text{ min}$$

Finally, calculate how many drops are required per minute:

$$\frac{7800 \text{ drops}}{300 \text{ min}} = 26 \text{ drops per minute.}$$

Example 14.18
A neonate weighing 3.0 kg is prescribed an infusion of phenytoin 15 mg/kg in normal saline for febrile convulsions. A giving set delivering 20 drops per minute is available. Recommend how this infusion should take place.

Phenytoin injection contains 50 mg/mL. The BNF indicates that the dose is 15–20 mg/kg in neonates at a rate of 1–3 mg/kg/min. The BNF also indicates that it is normal to use 50–100 mL of normal saline in such an infusion, so that the final concentration does not exceed 10 mg/mL. The total dose of phenytoin at 15 mg/kg is in line with the BNF recommendation. The amount of phenytoin required is $15 \times 3.0 = 45$ mg. Therefore, the volume of phenytoin injection required is $\frac{45}{50} = 0.90$ mL.

If this is added to 50 mL of normal saline it produces a volume of $50 + 0.9 = 50.9$ mL. The concentration is, therefore, $\frac{45}{50.9} = 0.88$ mg/mL. This concentration does not exceed the maximum recommended by the BNF.

The recommended rate of administration is 1–3 mg/kg/min. Taking the midpoint of 2 mg/kg/min, this converts to $2 \times 3.0 = 6$ mg/min. We now have a solution containing 0.88 mg/mL and a requirement of 6 mg/min. Therefore, the required rate is $\frac{6}{0.88} = 6.82$ mL/min.

The giving set has 20 drops per millilitre, therefore the number of drops per minute is $6.82 \times 20 = 136.4$ drops per minute. Therefore, it is suggested that a drop rate of 136 drops per minute be used to administer the 50.9 mL phenytoin infusion.

TOTAL PARENTERAL NUTRITION

Some patients are not able to take nutrition orally. When this is a long-term problem it is necessary to give all nutrients to the patient parenterally, a process referred to as total parenteral nutrition (TPN). A typical TPN solution will contain water and sources of protein, energy, electrolytes, trace elements, vitamins and minerals. They are, therefore, complex mixtures, which may have some problems with incompatibilities. More details about TPN mixtures can be found in reference sources such as *Pharmaceutical Practice* (3rd edition). The BNF includes a table of the proprietary infusion fluids used in TPN including the energy content and the quantity of potassium, magnesium, sodium, acetate and chloride ions, together with any other significant components. It should be noted that the ionic concentrations are given in mmol/L. Indeed prescriptions for TPN are normally written using mmol. The calculation of the amounts of the various ingredients to be included in an individual TPN mixture is usually performed in specialized units using computer programs which can also control the addition of the actual ingredients into the mixture.

It is outside the scope of this book to cover the processes in detail. Many of the calculations follow the patterns already illustrated in this and earlier chapters. However, two examples are included to illustrate the nature of some of the different calculations which can arise.

Example 14.19

A postoperative surgical patient requires 0.2 g/kg/24 h of nitrogen. The patient weighs 47 kg.

First, calculate the nitrogen requirements per 24 hours = 0.2×47 = 9.4 g nitrogen.

This requirement can then be matched up to commercially available amino acid solutions which are listed in the BNF.

Each gram of amino acid nitrogen is equivalent to 6.25 g of protein. For example, Vamin 9 contains 9.4 g/L of nitrogen. This is equivalent to nearly 60 g of protein and will provide the patient with the required daily nitrogen intake. However, care must also be taken when selecting an amino acid solution for inclusion in a TPN formulation, as most commercially available solutions are hypertonic and have a pH between 5 and 7.4. The pH of the amino acid solution may have an effect on the overall stability of the formulation and must be considered carefully.

Example 14.20

How many kilojoules does a patient receive from an infusion of 1 L of 10% dextrose? What volume of this infusion is required to provide 1200 kilojoules of energy to the patient? (One gram of dextrose provides 16 kilojoules of energy.)

First, calculate the weight of dextrose being administered in 1 litre. Therefore:

$$\frac{1000 \times 10}{100} = 100 \text{ g of dextrose}$$

The energy supplied is $100 \times 16 = 1600$ kJ. The volume of infusion required to provide 1200 kJ is obtained by simple proportion. Let the volume required be y. Therefore:

$$\frac{1000}{1600} = \frac{y}{1200} \text{ and } y = \frac{1000 \times 1200}{1600} = 750 \text{ mL}$$

An infusion of 750 mL will provide the patient with 1200 kJ of energy.

SELF-STUDY QUESTIONS

Depression of freezing point by a 1% w/v solution of sodium chloride is 0.576°C

14.1 Calculate how many mg of sodium chloride are required to make the following solutions isotonic:

(a) 50 mL of 2% pilocarpine hydrochloride. Depression of freezing point of a 1% solution is 0.134°C.

(b) 100 mL of 0.7% neomycin sulphate. Depression of freezing point of a 1% solution is 0.067°C.

(c) 150 mL of 0.5% chloramphenicol. Depression of freezing point of a 1% solution is 0.06°C.

14.2 Calculate how many mg of sodium chloride are required to make the following eye drops isotonic:

(a) 5 mL of 1% rose bengal. Depression of freezing point of a 1% solution is 0.040°C.

(b) 20 mL of 0.5% adrenaline hydrochloride (epinephrine hydrochloride). Depression of freezing point of a 1% solution is 0.165°C.

(c) 10 mL of 4% lidocaine hydrochloride (lignocaine hydrochloride). Depression of freezing point of a 1% solution is 0.125°C.

(d) 20 mL of 0.5% chloramphenicol. Depression of freezing point of a 1% solution is 0.06°C.

(e) 5 mL of 3% pilocarpine hydrochloride. Depression of freezing point of a 1% solution is 0.134°C.

(f) 10 mL of 2% fluorescein sodium. Depression of freezing point of a 1% solution is 0.182°C.

(g) 10 mL of 0.5% antazoline phosphate. Depression of freezing point of a 1% solution is 0.112°C.

(h) 15 mL of 0.3% gentamycin sulphate. Depression of freezing points of a 1% solution is 0.030°C.

(i) 10 mL of 0.25% timolol maleate. Depression of freezing point of a 1% solution is 0.077°C.

14.3 How much sodium chloride is required to make 150 mL of 0.25% zinc sulphate eye lotion isotonic? Depression of freezing point of a 1% solution is 0.085°C.

14.4 Calculate the amount of sodium chloride required to make the following eye lotion isotonic: zinc sulphate 0.3%, boric acid 0.75%, to 250 mL. Depressions of freezing point of 1% solutions: zinc sulphate 0.085°C, boric acid 0.283°C.

14.5 What weight of sodium chloride is required to make 20 mL of the following eye drops isotonic: cocaine hydrochloride 1.0%, homatropine hydrobromide 2.0%? Depressions of freezing point of 1% solutions: cocaine hydrochloride 0.091°C, homatropine hydrobromide 0.096°C.

14.6 Calculate the amount of sodium chloride required to make 100 mL of the following injection isotonic: ascorbic acid 1.0%, sodium bicarbonate 0.5%. Depressions of freezing point of 1% solutions: sodium bicarbonate 0.381°C, ascorbic acid 0.105°C.

14.7 The following infusions are to be made isotonic. Calculate the amount of sodium chloride required for each one:

(a) A patient weighing 132 lb is to receive an infusion of 75 mg/kg benzylpenicillin sodium in 500 mL of water. Depression of freezing point by a 1% solution is 0.100°C.

(b) A patient weighing 180 lb is to receive an infusion of 200 mg/kg benzylpenicillin sodium in 500 mL of water. Depression of freezing point by a 1% solution is 0.100°C.

(c) A patient weighing 60 kg is to receive an infusion of 30 mg/kg bretylium tosilate in 500 mL of water. Depression of freezing point by a 1% solution is 0.081°C.

(d) A patient weighing 154 lb is to receive an infusion of 12 mg/kg chloroquine phosphate in 500 mL of water. Depression of freezing point by a 1% solution is 0.082°C.

(e) A patient weighing 44 lb is to receive an infusion of 0.6 mg/kg chlorpromazine hydrochloride in 500 mL of water. Depression of freezing point by a 1% solution is 0.058°C.

(f) A patient weighing 132 lb is to receive an infusion of 12.5 mg/kg amikacin in 500 mL of water. Depression of freezing point by a 1% solution is 0.031°C.

(g) A patient weighing 154 lb is to receive an infusion of 100 mg/kg chloramphenicol sodium succinate in 500 mL of water. Depression of freezing point by a 1% solution is 0.078°C.

14.8 Calculate the volume of solution required to be added to the infusion fluid to provide the required dose:

(a) An injection of amphotericin containing 50 mg/10 mL to 500 mL of normal saline infusion to provide a total dose of 22 mg.

(b) An injection of polymyxin B sulphate containing 500 000 units/10 mL to 500 mL of normal saline infusion to produce a total dose of 97 500 units.

14.9 How much of the reconstituted injection should be added to the infusion fluid?

(a) An injection of aciclovir contains 250 mg/10 mL for addition to normal saline to produce 500 mL of 10 mg/mL infusion.

(b) An injection of amphotericin contains 5 mg/mL for addition to normal saline to produce 500 mL of 8 mg/10 mL infusion.

(c) An injection of colistin contains 500 000 units/mL for addition to normal saline to produce 500 mL of 105 000 units/mL infusion.

(d) An injection of aztreonam contains 125 mg/mL for addition to normal saline to produce 500 mL of 4 mg/mL infusion.

(e) An injection vial contains 500 mg of aciclovir to be reconstituted to 20 mL for addition to 500 mL of normal saline infusion to produce a 1.5 mg/mL solution.

(f) An injection vial contains 1 million units of colistin to be reconstituted to 20 mL for addition to 500 mL of infusion to contain 1050 units/mL.

(g) An injection vial contains 500 mg of aztreonam to be reconstituted to 4 mL for addition to 500 mL of normal saline infusion to produce a 2.5 mg/mL solution.

14.10 In preparing an IV infusion, you have a concentrated injection solution. What volume of this solution must be added to produce a 500 mL infusion with the required total dose?

(a) Adrenaline hydrochloride (epinephrine hydrochloride) (molecular weight 219.7) 1 g/mL to provide 15 mmol.

(b) Furosemide (frusemide) (molecular weight 330.7) 2 g/mL to provide 12 mmol.

(c) Erythromycin (molecular weight 733.9) 2 g/mL to provide 15 mmol.

(d) Cefotaxime sodium (molecular weight 477.4) 4 g/mL to provide 12 mmol.

(e) Cortisone (molecular weight 360.4) 2 g/mL to provide 10 mmol.

(f) Chloramphenicol (molecular weight 323.1) 2 g/mL to provide 20 mmol.

(g) Adrenaline acid tartrate (epinephrine bitartrate) (molecular weight 333.3) 3 g/mL to provide 10 mmol.

(h) Cefuroxime axetil (molecular weight 510.5) 2 g/mL to provide 20 mmol.

14.11 An infusion solution is available. What infusion rate (mL/min) should be used to provide the specified dosage rate? How long will the infusion last?

(a) 100 mg phenylephrine in 100 mL to give 130 µg/min

(b) 50 mg tacrolimus in 500 mL to give 50 µg/min

(c) 5 g bretylium tosilate in 500 mL to give 16 mg/min

14.12 For the following infusions, calculate the infusion rate (mL/min) and duration of infusion:

(a) An injection solution contains 1 mg/mL phenylephrine. 10 mL is added to 100 mL of 5% dextrose for infusion. The prepared infusion is to be administered at 40 µg/min.

(b) An injection solution contains 5 mg/mL tacrolimus. 5 mL is added to 50 mL of saline for infusion. The prepared infusion is to be administered at 2.5 mg/min.

(c) An injection solution contains 50 mg/mL bretylium tosilate. 3 mL is added to 60 mL of saline for infusion. The prepared infusion is to be administered at 1.6 mg/min.

14.13 A patient will receive an infusion using an infusion pump set at a particular value. What volume of infusion will he receive in the first time interval, and how long will it take to administer the total volume?

(a) Pump set to deliver 1 mL/min. Volume in the first 135 min and time for 500 mL.

(b) Pump set to deliver 45 mL/hour. Volume in the first 100 min and time for 500 mL.

(c) Pump set to deliver 30 mL/hour. Volume in the first 150 min and time for 250 mL.

(d) Pump set to deliver 75 mL/hour. Volume in the first 135 min and time for 500 mL.

14.14 For each infusion, calculate the infusion rate (mL/min) and, where appropriate, the duration of infusion before a replacement bag will be required.

(a) An infusion contains 2 mg/mL lidocaine hydrochloride (lignocaine hydrochloride) in 500 mL 5% glucose solution. The patient is to receive 4 mg/min for 30 minutes, followed by 2 mg/min for 2 hours, then 1 mg/min.

(b) An injection solution contains 10 mg/mL flecainide. 150 mL is added to 500 mL of saline for infusion. The patient, who weighs 70 kg, is to receive 1.5 mg/kg/h for 1 hour, then 200 µg/kg/h for 24 hours.

(c) An injection solution contains 20 mg/mL lidocaine hydrochloride (lignocaine hydrochloride). 20 mL are added to 500 mL of 5% glucose solution. The patient is to receive an infusion of 4 mg/min for 30 minutes, followed by 2 mg/min for 2 hours, then 1 mg/min.

14.15   An injection solution contains 10 mg/mL disopyramide. 5 mL is added to 100 mL of saline for infusion. The patient, who weighs 60 kg, is to receive 400 µg/kg/h. What rate of infusion should be used?

14.16   A specified giving set is to be used. What volume of infusion will the patient receive after the specified times?

(a) A patient is to receive a 5% dextrose infusion using a giving set delivering 40 mL/h. What volume in 30 minutes, 4 hours, 12 hours?

(b) A patient is to receive a 0.9% saline infusion using a giving set delivering 50 mL/h. What volume in 90 minutes, 150 minutes, 300 minutes?

(c) A patient is to receive a 5% dextrose infusion using a giving set delivering 65 mL/h. What volume in 60 minutes, 2.5 hours, 4 hours?

(d) A patient is to receive a 0.9% saline infusion using a giving set delivering 45 mL/h. What volume in 80 minutes, 170 minutes, 250 minutes?

14.17   What delivery rate (in mL/min) should be set on the infusion pump?

(a) 500 mL of 5% dextrose to be administered over 4 hours.

(b) 500 mL of 5% dextrose to be administered over 6 hours.

14.18   500 mL of 5% dextrose is to be administered over 360 minutes. What delivery rate should be set on the infusion pump? The infusion starts at 9 a.m. At what time will it be complete?

14.19 A patient will receive a saline infusion using an infusion pump, which is set to deliver 50 mL/h. How long would it take to administer 500 mL? If the infusion is started at 10 p.m., when will a new bag be required?

14.20 A patient will receive an infusion using an infusion pump, which is set to deliver 25 mL/h. How much fluid will the patient receive in the first 150 minutes? When will a 250 mL infusion be complete if it is started at 2.30 p.m.?

14.21 A patient will receive an infusion using an infusion pump, which is set to deliver 75 mL/h. The infusion starts at 11 a.m. At what time will 500 mL have been administered?

14.22 What rate, in mL/min, should be used to administer these infusions?

(a) 10 mL of a solution containing 500 mg of cefatoxime is added to 100 mL of 5% dextrose infusion for administration over 60 minutes.
(b) 10 mL of a solution containing 100 mg of metaraminol is added to 500 mL of 5% dextrose infusion for administration over 5 hours.
(c) 20 mL of a solution containing 15 000 units of bleomycin is added to 200 mL of saline infusion for administration over 3 hours.
(d) 2 mL of a solution containing 500 mg of amikacin sulphate is added to 100 mL of saline infusion for administration over 0.5 hour.

14.23 What volume of diluent is required to complete the infusion solution and what rate of infusion is required?

(a) A 250 mL intravenous solution of foscarnet sodium contains 24 mg/mL. This is to be diluted to produce 12 mg/mL in 5% glucose and administered over 2 hours.
(b) 1 g of erythromycin lactobionate is dissolved in 20 mL of saline. It must be diluted to give a concentration of 5 mg/mL and then administered over 60 minutes.

14.24 For each infusion, how many drops/min should be administered?

(a) 10 mL of a solution containing 500 mg of cefotaxime is added to 500 mL of 5% dextrose infusion for administration over 5 hours using a 'giving set' which provides 10 drops/mL.

(b) 10 mL of a solution containing 500 mg of cefatoxime is added to 500 mL of 5% dextrose infusion for administration over 10 hours using a 'giving set' which provides 20 drops/mL.

(c) 20 mL of a solution containing 15 000 units of bleomycin is added to 500 mL of saline infusion for administration over 3 hours using a 'giving set' which provides 20 drops/mL.

(d) 15 mL of a solution containing 500 mg of rituximab is added to 500 mL of saline infusion for administration over 8 hours using a 'giving set' which provides 60 drops/mL.

(e) 15 mL of a solution containing 500 mg of rituximab is added to 500 mL of saline infusion for administration over 5 hours using a 'giving set' which provides 15 drops/mL.

14.25 A 250 mL intravenous solution of foscarnet sodium contains 24 mg/mL. This is to be diluted to produce 12 mg/mL in 5% glucose and administered over 3 hours. What volume is required to complete the infusion solution? Using a giving set delivering 20 drops/mL, how many drops/min should be the rate of administration?

14.26 What rate, in drops/min, should be administered using a 20 drops/mL giving set?

(a) 10 mL of a solution containing 100 mg of metaraminol is added to 500 mL of 5% dextrose infusion for administration over 5 hours.

(b) 2 mL of a solution containing 500 mg of amikacin sulphate is added to 100 mL of saline infusion for administration over 0.5 hour.

(c) 1 g of erythromycin lactobionate is dissolved in 20 mL saline. It must be diluted to give a concentration of 10 mg/mL and then administered over 60 minutes.

14.27 An infusion solution contains 100 mg phenylephrine in 500 mL. What rate of infusion should be used to give 130 µg/min when using a giving set delivering 20 drops/mL?

14.28 50 mg of sodium nitroprusside has been diluted to 1000 mL in 5% glucose infusion. It is to be administered to a 78 kg patient at a rate of 0.8 µg/kg/min for 5 minutes, and then will be increased by 500 ng/kg/min each 5 minutes to a maximum of 15 minutes. Calculate the infusion rates required. What would be the drop rate if a 60 drops/mL giving set is used?

For answers to these questions see page 291

15 Other practice related topics

After studying this chapter you will be able to:

- Arrive at a value for body mass index for an individual
- Carry out simple pharmacoeconomic calculations in connection with the cost and benefit of given drug treatments
- Calculate the costs of medicines to be provided by sale or on private prescription allowing for discounts, markups and professional fees

BODY MASS INDEX (BMI)

Being overweight increases the risk for many chronic conditions such as coronary heart disease (CHD), hypertension and type 2 diabetes mellitus. However, being grossly overweight or obese predisposes the patient to a greater risk of chronic conditions, disease complications and mortality. To prevent this risk, pharmacists routinely advise patients on general maintenance of good health, and provide counselling with regard to weight control. Weight control may be achieved by dietary therapy, adequate exercise, pharmacotherapy, and, in extreme cases of obesity, weight loss surgery.

To commence the management of obese patients, an assessment is made of the BMI which is a clinical standard for judging excessive weight. Simply, BMI is the body weight in kilograms divided by the square of height measured in metres. Individuals with a BMI of 30 and above are considered obese, whereas those with a BMI between 18.5 and 29.9 may be considered weight-normal.

Calculations of body mass index (BMI)

Example 15.1
Calculate the body mass index of a patient 5 feet 2 inches and weighing 96 pounds.

The equivalents are: 2.2 lb = 1 kg, and 39.37 in = 1 metre (m).
Let y be the weight in kg:

$$\frac{96 \text{ lb}}{2.2 \text{ lb}} = \frac{y \text{ kg}}{1 \text{ kg}}, \text{ therefore } y = \frac{96 \times 1}{2.2} = 43.64 \text{ kg}$$

Let z be the height in m:

$$\frac{[(5 \times 12) + 2 \text{ in}]}{39.37 \text{ in}} = \frac{z}{1 \text{ m}}, \text{ therefore } z = \frac{62 \times 1}{39.37} = 1.57 \text{ m}$$

$$\text{BMI} = \frac{\text{weight (kg)}}{\text{height (m}^2)} = \frac{43.64 \text{ kg}}{(1.57 \text{ m} \times 1.57 \text{ m})} = \frac{43.64 \text{ kg}}{2.46 \text{ m}^2} = 17.7 = 18 \text{ BMI}$$

Example 15.2
Calculate the BMI of a patient 6 feet 3 inches in height weighing 180 lb.

$$\frac{180 \text{ lb}}{2.2 \text{ lb}} = \frac{y \text{ kg}}{1 \text{ kg}}, y = 81.82 \text{ kg, and } \frac{75 \text{ in}}{39.37 \text{ in}} = \frac{z}{1 \text{ m}}, z = 1.91 \text{ m}$$

$$\text{BMI} = \frac{81.82 \text{ kg}}{1.91 \text{ m} \times 1.91 \text{ m}} = \frac{81.82 \text{ kg}}{3.65 \text{ m}^2} = 22.4 = 22 \text{ BMI}$$

Determining BMI from a standardized table

The body mass index (BMI) of a person may be determined from a standardized table as shown in Table 15.1, in which the intercept of the height and weight indicates the BMI.

Example 15.3
Determine the BMI from Table 15.1 for a person 5 feet 3 inches in height and weighing 130 lb.

The intercept of 5 ft 3 in in height and 130 lb shows a BMI of 23.

Example 15.4
Using Table 15.1, determine the BMI for a patient 180 cm in height and weighing 78 kg.

Since Table 15.1 is in feet/inches and pounds, the height of the patient is converted to inches and the weight to pounds:

Table 15.1 Determining Body Mass Index (BMI) from a standardized table

Weight (lb)

Height	100	110	120	130	140	150	160	170	180	190	200	210	220	230	240	250
5'0"	20	21	23	25	27	29	31	33	35	37	39	41	43	45	47	48
5'1"	19	21	23	25	25	28	30	32	34	36	38	40	42	43	45	47
5'2"	18	20	22	24	25	27	29	31	33	35	37	39	40	42	44	46
5'3"	18	19	21	23	25	27	28	30	32	34	35	37	38	41	43	44
5'4"	17	19	21	22	24	26	27	29	31	33	34	35	38	38	41	43
5'5"	17	18	20	22	23	25	27	28	30	32	33	35	37	38	40	42
5'6"	16	18	19	21	23	24	26	27	29	31	32	34	36	37	39	40
5'7"	16	17	19	20	22	23	25	27	28	30	31	33	34	36	38	39
5'8"	15	17	18	20	21	23	24	26	27	29	30	32	33	35	36	38
5'9"	15	16	18	19	21	22	24	25	27	28	30	31	32	34	35	37
5'10"	14	16	17	19	20	22	23	24	26	27	29	30	32	33	34	36
5'11"	14	15	17	18	20	21	22	24	25	26	28	29	30	32	33	35
6'0"	14	15	16	18	19	20	22	23	24	26	27	28	30	31	33	34
6'1"	13	15	16	17	18	20	21	22	24	25	26	28	29	30	32	33
6'2"	13	14	15	17	18	19	21	22	23	24	25	27	28	30	31	32
6'3"	12	14	15	16	17	19	20	21	22	24	25	26	27	29	30	31
6'4"	12	13	15	16	17	18	19	21	22	23	24	26	27	28	29	30

BMI interpretation: Underweight: under 18.51. Normal: 18.5–24. Overweight: 25–29.9. Obese: 30 and over.

$$\frac{180 \text{ cm}}{2.54 \text{ cm}} = \frac{y \text{ in}}{1 \text{ in}}, \text{ therefore } y = \frac{180 \times 1}{2.54} = 71 \text{ in} = 5 \text{ ft } 11 \text{ in}$$

$$\frac{78 \text{ kg}}{1 \text{ kg}} = \frac{z \text{ lb}}{2.2 \text{ lb}}, \text{ therefore } z = \frac{78 \times 2.2}{1} = 172 \text{ lb.}$$

The intercept of 5 ft 11 in in height and 170 lb shows a BMI of 24.

PHARMACOECONOMIC CALCULATIONS

Pharmacoeconomic calculations deal with the economic aspects of drugs, and costs of drug therapy analysed against therapeutic outcomes. Also considered in pharmacoeconomics are drug product acquisition costs at retail and consumer levels; inventory, financial and human resource management, cost versus benefit relationships of drug therapy decisions, non-drug treatment alternatives, and health outcomes; drug product selection and drug formulary decisions; impact of proper drug utilization on incidence of hospitalization and length of stay; economic and health consequences of patient noncompliance, drug misuse, and adverse drug reactions. Further information is available in *Pharmaceutical Practice* (3rd edition). The following are introductory calculations that exemplify the general methods of pharmacoeconomic analysis, cost differentials related to drug product selection, drug acquisition costs and dispensing fees.

Cost–benefit analysis

Cost–benefit analysis determines all of the costs of providing a programme or treatment and compares these costs with the benefits that result.

$$\text{Benefit to cost ratio} = \frac{\text{benefit (£)}}{\text{costs (£)}}$$

If the result is a number greater than '1', the benefits exceed the costs and the treatment is considered beneficial.

Example 15.5

Calculate the benefit to cost ratio for a programme in which the cost of a pharmacist intervention was £24 000 and the benefits accrued were £50 000.

$$\text{Benefit to cost ratio} = \frac{\text{benefits (£)}}{\text{costs (£)}} = \frac{\text{£50 000}}{\text{£ 24 000}} = 2.1$$

Cost–effectiveness analysis

Cost-effectiveness analysis is used for comparing the cost of treatment alternatives (measured in currency) and the treatment outcomes expressed in terms of the therapeutic objective (such as lowering of blood pressure). This is expressed as the cost to effectiveness ratio (C/E ratio):

$$\text{Cost to effectiveness ratio} = \frac{\text{Costs (£)}}{\text{Therapeutic effects (in measurable units)}}$$

Example 15.6

Determine the cost to effectiveness ratios for two 12-month treatments for lowering systolic blood pressure. Treatment A cost £2400 and lowered systolic blood pressure by an average of 5 mm of mercury. Treatment B cost £1600 and lowered systolic blood pressure by an average of 8 mm of mercury.

Treatment A

$$\text{C/E ratio} = \frac{\text{£2400}}{5 \, \text{mm Hg}} = 480 \, (\text{£/mm Hg}).$$

Treatment B

$$\text{C/E ratio} = \frac{\text{£1600}}{8 \, \text{mm Hg}} = 200 \, (\text{£/mm Hg})$$

Therefore Treatment B has a better cost to effectiveness ratio.

Cost–minimization analysis

Cost–minimization analysis deals with the comparison of two or more treatment alternatives, the outcomes of which are assumed or determined to be equivalent. The cost of each treatment alternative is expressed in currency terms and the costs compared.

Example 15.7

In a diabetes clinic, cost–minimization analyses determined that two alternative treatments cost £2240 (Treatment C) and £2900 (Treatment D) respectively. What is the cost benefit of Treatment C compared to Treatment D?

Cost benefit = Treatment D – Treatment C = £2900 – £2240 = £660

Cost differential between therapeutic agents

In general, newer drugs within a therapeutic class are more expensive than older agents because of innovation and the cost of production of the new drugs. So there can be a substantial cost difference between drugs within the same therapeutic class. Therefore, therapeutic interchange programs, which allow for the substitution of one drug over another while maintaining comparable therapeutic benefit, can result in cost savings.

Example 15.8

Calculate the cost differential between the thrombolytic agents streptokinase (500 000 IU costs £28.66) and the biotechnology derived alteplase (100 mg costs £600.00) if the total amount required to be administered to a patient is either 3000 000 IU of streptokinase or 180 mg of alteplase.

Let y be the cost of streptokinase:

$$\frac{3000\ 000\ \text{IU}}{500\ 000\ \text{IU}} = \frac{y}{£28.66}, \text{ therefore } y = \frac{3000\ 000 \times 28.66}{500\ 000} = £171.96$$

Let z be the cost of alteplase:

$$\frac{180\ \text{mg}}{100\ \text{mg}} = \frac{z}{£600.00}, \text{ therefore } z = \frac{180 \times 600.00}{100} = £1080.00$$

Cost differential is £1080.00 – £171.96 = £908.04.

Cost differential between branded drugs and generic equivalents

Brand-name drug products are generally more expensive than generic equivalents, and decisions on selecting a certain drug product may be made on cost basis by health care providers.

Example 15.9

A brand-name drug costs $92.40/100 tablets while the generic equivalent costs $24.80/100 tablets. Calculate the drug cost differential for a 30-day supply if a patient takes two tablets daily.

Tablets needed at 2 tablets (daily) × 30 (days) = 60 tablets.
Let y be the cost of generic drug:

$$\frac{60 \text{ tablets}}{100 \text{ tablets}} = \frac{y}{\$24.80}, \text{ therefore } y = \frac{60 \times 24.80}{100} = \$14.88$$

Let z be the cost of branded drug:

$$\frac{60 \text{ tablets}}{100 \text{ tablets}} = \frac{z}{\$92.40}, \text{ therefore } z = \frac{60 \times 92.40}{100} = \$55.44$$

Therefore, the cost differential = $55.44 – $14.88 = $40.56.

Cost differential between dosage forms and routes of administration

Generally, tablets and capsules are less expensive to manufacture than injectable products. Therefore, a cost differential is likely to exist between dosage forms of the same therapeutic agent due to the costs of production. For patients on intravenous therapy, there are additional personnel and equipment needed to administer the medication. Thus, it is desirable to encourage the conversion of parenteral medications to oral therapy without compromising the desired therapeutic outcomes.

Example 15.10

Verapamil 80 mg tablets are taken three times a day and cost £2.50/100 tablets. Extended release capsules containing 240 mg of verapamil are taken once daily and cost £12.24/28 capsules. Calculate the treatment cost differential over a 30-day period.

Cost per 80 mg tablet: £2.50/100 (tablets) = £0.025 (per tablet).
3 tablets (per day) × 30 (days) = 90 tablets are required.
Therefore total cost is £0.025 × 90 (tablets) = £2.25.
Cost per 240 mg capsule: £12.24/28 (capsules) = £0.437 (per capsule).
1 capsule (per day) × 30 (days) = 30 capsules.
Therefore total cost is £0.437 × 30 (capsules) = £13.11.
Cost differential is £13.11 – £2.25 = £10.86 per 30-day course.

Example 15.11

A patient was switched from intravenous ciprofloxacin (400 mg
12 hourly) to oral ciprofloxacin (500 mg 12 hourly). Calculate the daily
drug savings if the intravenous product costs € (euro)1.20 per 200 mg
and the oral product costs € 0.30 per 250 mg capsule.

Every 12 hours is twice daily.

Intravenous ciprofloxacin requires 400 mg × 2 = 800 mg daily. This
costs:

$$\frac{800 \text{ mg} \times € 1.20}{200 \text{ mg}} = € 4.80.$$

Oral ciprofloxacin requires 500 mg × 2 = 1000 mg daily. This costs:

$$\frac{1000 \text{ mg} \times € 0.30}{250 \text{ mg}} = € 1.20.$$

Thus, the cost differential is € 4.80 – € 1.20 = € 3.60 per day.

Cost differential of dosing regimen

A dosing regimen for a specific drug may be changed to be
more cost-effective without affecting the desired therapeutic
outcome.

Example 15.12

A dosage interval adjustment was made for ranitidine in a group of 46
hospitalized patients so that the number of doses per patient per
treatment day was reduced from an average of 2.00 to 1.00 without
sacrificing therapeutic outcomes. If the cost of each dose of ranitidine
was £0.27, calculate the daily cost savings to the hospital.

Reduction in doses per patient per day is (2.00 – 1.00) = 1.00 dose.
Reduction in doses in the whole patient group is 1.00 dose × 46 =
46 doses.

Therefore the total cost saving is £0.27 × 46 doses = £12.42 per day.

Cost differential of alternative treatment plans

Non-pharmacological approaches, exercises, preventive
medicine, drug therapy, physiotherapy, electroconvulsive
therapy, radiation and surgery are valid alternatives in
maintaining health, or in treating diseased conditions.

Example 15.13
If the daily treatment of an epileptic patient with phenytoin prevents readmission to a hospital, calculate the potential savings over hospitalization if the daily drug costs are £0.85 and the average 5-day hospital bill was £2056.

Drug cost: £0.85 × 5 (days) = £4.25
Potential savings is the difference between the two costs:

Hospitalization − drug treatment = £2056 − £4.25 = £2051.75

DRUG ACQUISITION COSTS

Pharmacists buy medications and other merchandise from wholesalers and manufacturers, and may get discounts based on quantity purchased, prompt payment of invoices, or for certain seasonal products. These discounts provide the pharmacy with a means of increasing the gross profit on certain products. Therefore, the actual acquisition cost for a given product is the list price, less all discounts that are applied.

Calculating net cost when given list price and allowable discount

The net cost of a medication is the list price less the allowable discount.

Example 15.14
The list price of a cough syrup is £3.50 per 500 mL, less 40% discount. What is the net cost per 500 mL of the cough syrup?

Net cost = list price − discount = 100% − 40% = 60%.

Therefore: net cost = £3.50 × 60/100 = £2.10

Calculating net cost when given list price and a series of discounts

Several discounts may be allowed on promotional deals. For example, the list price on paracetamol tablets may be subject to a trade discount of 30%, plus a quantity discount of 10% and a cash discount of 4% for prompt payment of the invoice. This chain of deductions, called a *series discount*, may be converted to a single discount equivalent. The discounts in the series cannot be calculated by adding them; rather the first discount is deducted from the list price and each successive discount is taken on the balance remaining after deduction of the preceding discount. The order in which the discounts in a series discount are taken is not important.

Example 15.15

The list price of 20 bottles each containing100 antipyretic tablets is £72.00, less a trade discount of 35%. If purchased in quantities of 12 dozens, an additional discount of 12% is allowed by the manufacturer, plus a 4% cash discount for payment of the invoice within 7 days of billing. Calculate the net cost of 144 bottles of the antipyretic tablets when purchased under the conditions of the offer.

List price of 20 bottles = £72.00.

List price of 144 = $\dfrac{£72 \times 144}{20}$ = £518.40.

Discounts: 100% − 35% = 65%; 100% − 12% = 88%;
100% − 4% = 96%.
Cost after 35% is deducted is £518.40 × 65% = £336.96.
Cost after 12% is deducted is £336.96 × 88% = £296.52.
Cost after 4% is deducted is £296.52 × 96% = £284.66.

Single discount equivalent for a series of discounts

To calculate a single discount equivalent to a series of discounts, subtract each discount from 100% and multiply the net percentages together. The product obtained is subtracted from 100% to give the single discount equivalent to the series discount. For instance, a company may introduce a new brand of antidiabetic medication to the market. To encourage pharmacists to stock it, the company may give a trade discount of 30% for purchasing large quantities, an off invoice allowance of 15% for making payment within two weeks of receiving the invoice, and a display allowance of 8% for placing the product on the shelves for patients to see and purchase.

Example 15.16

The special sale of pharmaceuticals gives a trade discount of 30%, an off invoice allowance of 15%, and a display allowance of 8%. What is the single discount equivalent to these discounts?

Individual discounts are: 100% − 30% = 70%; 100% − 15% = 85%; 100% − 8% = 92%.

Percentage to be paid: $\dfrac{70}{100} \times \dfrac{85}{100} \times \dfrac{92}{100} = 54.7\%$.

Single discount equivalent = 100% − 54.7% = 45.3%.

Mark-up

Mark-up (or the margin of profit) is the difference between the cost of an item and its selling price. For instance, if a pharmacist buys a bottle of elixir for £2.00 and sells it for £3.20, the mark-up (or gross profit) is £1.20. Mark-up percent (percent of gross profit) is the mark-up divided by the selling price expressed as a percentage. It expresses the percentage that the mark-up is of the selling price.

Example 15.17

The cost of 100 anticonvulsant tablets is € 42.00. What should a pharmacist make the selling price to yield a 60% gross profit on the cost?

Gross profit = cost × % of gross profit = € 42.00 × 60% = € 25.20

Selling price = cost + gross profit = € 42.00 + € 25.20 = € 67.20.

Example 15.18

The cost of 100 anticonvulsant tablets is € 42.00. What should a pharmacist make the selling price to yield a 33% gross profit on the selling price?

Selling price = 100%:

Selling price − gross profit = cost price; 100% − 33% = 67%

Let y be the selling price:

$\dfrac{\text{Cost price}}{\text{Selling price}} = \dfrac{67\%}{100\%} = \dfrac{€\ 42.00}{y}$, therefore $y = \dfrac{€\ 42.00 \times 100}{67} = €\ 62.69$.

Example 15.19

What should the percent mark-up on the cost of an item be to yield a 30% gross profit on the selling price?

Selling price = 100%:

Cost = selling price – gross profit; 100% – 30% = 70%

Let y be the percentage gross profit on the cost:

$$\frac{\text{Cost as \% of selling price}}{\text{Selling price as \%}} = \frac{\text{gross profit as \% of selling price}}{y\ (\%)}$$

Thus, $\frac{70\%}{100\%} = \frac{30\%}{y\%}$, therefore, $y\% = \frac{30 \times 100}{70} = 42.86\%$.

PRESCRIPTION PRICING

Prescription pricing is a process of determining the amount of money that a patient pays when a private prescription (i.e. not National Health Service in the UK) was written by the prescriber and is dispensed in a pharmacy. It ensures a reasonable profit that enables the pharmacy to provide services to the patient and the community. The methods of prescription pricing include the following:

Percent mark-up

A desired percentage increase on the cost of the ingredients is added to the cost of the ingredients to obtain the prescription price.

Prescription price = (cost of ingredients × % mark-up) + cost of ingredients.

Example 15.20

If the cost of a medication to be dispensed is £10.00 and the pharmacist applies 70% mark-up on cost, what would be the prescription price?

Prescription price = (£10.00 × 70%) + £10.00 = £7.00 + £10.00 = £17.00.

Percent mark-up plus professional fee

Both a percent mark-up and a professional fee are added to the cost of the ingredients to obtain the prescription price. The professional fee is established to recover the combined cost of the container, overheads and counselling services.

Prescription price = (cost of ingredients × % mark-up) + cost of ingredients + fee.

Example 15.21
If the cost of a medication to be dispensed is £8.00 and the pharmacist applies a 20% mark-up on cost plus a professional fee of £4.50, what would be the prescription price?

(£8.00 × 20%) + £8.00 + £4.50 = £1.60 + £8.00 + £4.50 = £14.10.

Cost of medication plus professional fee

The prescription price is obtained by adding a professional fee to the cost of the medication. A true professional fee is independent of the cost of medication, and it does not change from one prescription to another. However, some pharmacists use a variable professional fee method whereby the amount of the fee varies depending on the cost of the medication. Pharmacies that charge a professional fee usually charge more for prescriptions requiring compounding to compensate for the extra time, ingredients and equipment used.

Example 15.22
If the cost of a medication to be dispensed is £8.00 and the pharmacist applies a professional fee of £8.50, what would be the prescription price?

Prescription price = cost of ingredients + professional fee

£8.00 + £8.50 = £16.50.

Average wholesale price (AWP)

Many government agencies and insurance companies use the professional fee method for the reimbursement of pharmacists in filling prescriptions under their programmes. Such third-party payers establish the professional fee to be adopted with pharmacists participating in the programmes. Since the actual cost of a medication varies between pharmacies, depending on the discounts received, most third party payers use the average wholesale price (AWP) less an established percentage as the cost basis for the medication in reimbursement programmes. The AWP is obtained from commercial listings, and the reimbursed amount is calculated from a predetermined formula, for example, 'AWP less 8% plus $9.00 professional fee'. In addition, many third-party programmes have a 'co-payment' provision which requires the patient to pay a portion of the charge for each prescription dispensed.

Example 15.23
If a third-party payer reimburses a pharmacy 'AWP less 8 %' plus a professional fee of £9.50, what would be the total reimbursement on a prescription calling for 48 capsules having an AWP of £50.00 per 100 capsules?

$$AWP = \frac{48 \times 50}{100} = £24.00.$$

$$Total\ reimbursement = £24.00 - \frac{(24 \times 8)}{100} + £9.50$$
$$= £22.08 + £9.50 = £31.58.$$

Example 15.24
If a pharmacy provider contract calls for a co-payment of £5.00 to be paid directly to the pharmacy for each prescription the patient has filled, how much would the third party reimburse the pharmacy in Example 15.23?

$$£31.58 - £5.00 = £26.58$$

Group health insurance coverage often provides reimbursement benefits only after a patient reaches a self-paid level (the stated 'deductible' amount) of his or her health care expenses, after which the coverage may pay fully or partially for certain covered expenses.

Example 15.25
Group health insurance covers 90% of prescription drug costs after a $500.00 deductible amount is reached. If, after making payments of

$475.00 toward the deductible amount, a patient pays a pharmacy $92.00 for a prescription, how much can he expect to be reimbursed by his insurance carrier?

$500.00 – $475.00 = $25.00 is remaining toward the deductible amount.
$92.00 – $25.00 = $67.00 is covered expense, therefore
$67.00 × 90% = $60.30 reimbursement is due.

SELF-STUDY QUESTIONS

15.1 Using the standardized BMI table (feet/inches and pounds), determine the BMI of a patient measuring 69 inches in height and weighing 140 pounds.

15.2 Calculate the BMI for a patient standing 5 feet 11 inches in height and weighing 190 pounds (round off answer to whole number).

15.3 Calculate the BMI for a person who is 1.9 m tall and weighs 109 kg (round off answer to whole number) and comment on the value.

15.4 By cost–benefit analysis, determine the numerical result of a programme in which pharmacist intervention costing £9000 resulted in benefits valued at £16 000.

15.5 An antihypertensive drug is available in a three-times-a-day tablet at £48.00/100 tablets, in a twice-a-day tablet at £72.00/100 tablets and in a once-a-day tablet at £96.00/100 tablets. Which form would be most economical to a compliant patient for a week's treatment and at what cost?

15.6 A pharmacist offers a patient the option of dispensing 30 scored atenolol 100 mg tablets (for the patient to break in half with a dose of one half tablet) or 60 tablets containing 50 mg of the drug. Calculate the cost differential and indicate the most economical option for the patient if the 100 mg tablets cost $96.00 per 100 tablets and the 50 mg tablets cost $93.00 per 100 tablets.

15.7 If 100 tablets of a brand name drug cost £200.00 and 60 tablets of a generic equivalent cost £30.00, calculate the differential cost of a 30-day treatment, if a patient is required to take one tablet daily.

15.8 The clinical pharmacist recommended parenteral cefazolin (dose: 0.5 g eight hourly; cost: £0.90/g) over parenteral cefoxitin (dose: 1 g six hourly; cost: £3.24/g) to balance therapeutic outcomes with cost containment. Calculate the difference in drug cost between these two treatments per day.

15.9 The medication hydralazine may be given intravenously when needed to control hypertension at 20 mg doses in 5% dextrose in water every 12 hours for 48 hours, after which the patient is converted to oral dosage, 10 mg tablets four times per day for 2 days, then 25 mg tablets four times per day for the next 5 days. If the 20 mg IV ampoule costs £1.54; 10 mg tablets, £2.31/100 tablets; 25 mg tablets, £2.70/100 tablets; 5% dextrose in water, £5.42/bottle.

15.10 The cost to a hospital of the drug diazepam is £1.06 per 10 mg vial. If the drug is administered by intravenous injection at 0.10 mg/kg/h for 24 hours, calculate the daily cost of the drug used for a 68 kg patient.

15.11 The intravenous dosing schedules and costs of the following cephalosporin antimicrobial agents are: cefazolin, 1 g every 8 hours (£4.63/g); cefoxitin, 1 g every 6 hours (£4.92/g) and cefotan, 1 g every 24 hours (£18.82/g). Compare the daily cost of each drug.

15.12 Calculate the single discount equivalent to each of the following series of deductions:
- **(a)** A trade discount of 35%, a quantity discount of 6% and a cash discount of 4%.
- **(b)** A trade discount of 30%, a 12% off invoice allowance, and additional 8% display allowance.
- **(c)** A trade discount of 38%, a display allowance of 9% and a cash discount of 5%.

15.13   A sunscreen lotion is listed at £26.18 per dozen 180 mL bottles, less a discount of 40%. The supplier offers two bottles free with the purchase of 10 on a promotional deal. What is the net cost per bottle when the lotion is purchased on the deal?

15.14   A pharmacist receives a bill of goods amounting to £600.00, less a 9% discount for quantity buying and a 4% cash discount for paying the invoice within 7 days. What is the net amount paid by the pharmacist?

15.15   A salbutamol inhaler costs £21.12 per dozen units, less a discount of 35%, plus an additional promotional discount of 8%. Calculate the net cost per unit.

15.16   Calculate the difference in the net cost of a bill of goods amounting to £5000 if the bill is discounted at single 35%, and if it is discounted at successive 28% and 9%.

15.17

℞

Belladonna Tincture 60 mL
Phenobarbital elixir ad 480 mL
Sig. 5 mL in water a.c.
Belladonna tincture costs £16.40/L, and the phenobarbital elixir was bought on a special deal at £26.80/5L, less 10%. Calculate the net cost of the ingredients for the prescription.

15.18   A brand of cleansing cream is sold for £3.75 per jar, thereby yielding a gross profit of 65% on the cost. How much did it cost?

15.19   One dozen tubes of lubricating jelly are listed at £15.00, with discounts of 20% and 10% when purchased in gross quantities. Calculate the net cost per tube.

15.20   Twelve bottles of 100 antihypertensive tablets cost £9.80 when bought on a promotional deal. If the tablets sell for £1.40 per 100, what percent of gross profit is realized on the selling price?

15.21   Twenty bottles of 1000 analgesic tablets are listed at £800.00 with discounts of 30% and 5%. At what price per 100 must the tablets be sold to yield a gross profit of 48% on the selling price?

15.22   A pharmacist sells a jar of cream for £7.50, thereby realizing a gross profit of 54% on the cost. Calculate the cost of the cream.

15.23   A bottle of lotion is listed at £1.00. Calculate the difference between a single discount of 32% and successive discounts of 20% and 12%.

15.24   A pharmacist sells a bottle of lotion for £4.88, to make a profit of 30% on the selling price. Calculate the cost of the lotion.

15.25   A pharmacist purchased 1 dozen bottles of an ophthalmic solution listed at € 36.00 per dozen. A discount of 40% was allowed on the purchase plus a 5% discount for paying the bill by the fifth day of the month. At what price per bottle would the solution be sold to give a gross profit of 30% on the selling price?

15.26   A prescription item costs a pharmacist £6.40. Using a mark-up of 40% on the cost, what would be the price of the dispensed prescription?

15.27   A pharmacist decided to determine a professional fee by calculating the average mark-up on a series of previously filled prescriptions. A sample of 200 prescriptions had a total cost to the pharmacist of £1120 and a total prescription price of £2172. Calculate the average professional fee that could be used in prescription pricing.

For answers to these questions see page 293

Basic statistics

After studying this chapter you will be able to understand
basic statistical concepts, and undertake calculations
dealing with:

- Mean, median and mode in a set of data
- Determination of standard deviation, and relative
  standard deviation
- Normal distribution, and confidence interval for a
  population mean
- Chi-squared test for association between two variables

Statistics may be defined as the science of collecting,
classifying and interpreting facts on the basis of relative
number or occurrence in order to make an inference. Thus, all
statistical studies begin with the gathering of data, and the
information, or 'raw data', is tabulated and analysed for
significance and validity by mathematical and graphical
procedures.

THE DATA

When numeric facts are collected, they are initially recorded in
any order. However, a logical arrangement of it must be made
for the data to be analysed effectively. The 'raw data' must be
tabulated, and this consists of listing the items in a set of
values or variables in order of magnitude, from smallest to
largest or largest to smallest. In this way, the data are
organized. For instance, a given set of data of patients'
temperatures (°C) can be tabulated from the lowest to the
highest:

Temperature (°C)

37.3	37.5	37.6	37.6	37.8
37.4	37.5	37.6	37.7	37.8
37.4	37.6	37.6	37.7	37.9
37.5	37.6	37.6	37.7	38.0

A better tabulation consists of arranging the given data in classes and listing their frequencies. Such an arrangement results in the *frequency distribution*. In this arrangement, the data are both organized and reduced. The frequency distribution of the patients' temperatures is made by placing the data into classes and writing the number of times a value appears in each class. If five classes of 0.2°C beginning with 37.15°C are chosen, the tabulation is made in the following manner:

Class (°C)	Tally	Frequency
37.15–37.35	|	1
37.35–37.55	ⅢⅢ	5
37.55–37.75	ⅢⅢ ⅢⅢ	10
37.75–37.95	|||	3
37.95–38.15	|	1
		Total: 20

The frequency distribution shows a concentration of data in the 37.55–37.75°C class. Generally, frequency distributions should have not less than five and not more than 15 classes. The choice of the number of classes depends on the nature of the data.

AVERAGES

Mean, median and mode

The *arithmetic mean* or *average* is a measure of central tendency. This measure is calculated by adding the values of all the items in a set of data and dividing by the number of items. The formula for the arithmetic mean or average is:

$$\bar{X} = \frac{\text{sum of values } (X)}{\text{number of values}} = \frac{\Sigma X}{n}$$

The notation $\bar{X}$ (read as x-bar) represents the average. The symbol Σ (the Greek capital letter sigma) means the summation of all the items of the variable X, and n refers to the number of values in the given set of data.

The average of the tabulated data on patients' temperatures can be calculated from the formula. Thus:

$$\text{Average} = \frac{1(37.3) + 2(37.4) + 3(37.5) + 7(37.6) + 3(37.7) + 2(37.8) + 1(37.9) + 1(38.0)}{20}$$

$$= \frac{752.4}{20} = 37.6°C$$

Another type of average is called the *median*. The median is also the *fiftieth percentile* of a distribution, i.e. the value below which 50% of the data is found. The median represents the *middle* item in a series; it is the middle item when there are an odd number of items. The median may be considered the average of the two middle items or, if greater precision is desired, it is the *weighted average* of the two middle items (tenth and eleventh in the data of patients' temperatures). From the data of the patients' temperatures, the median can be calculated. Thus:

$$\text{Average of the two middle temperatures} = \frac{37.6 + 37.6}{2}$$

$$= \frac{75.2}{2} = 37.6°C$$

A further type of summary measure is the *mode.*It is the item that appears most *frequently* in a set of data. The mode in the set of patients' temperatures is 37.6°C because that temperature appears the greatest number of times in the tabulation. The mode and the median are considered as 'positional averages' because they are determined by location. The arithmetic mean is a 'calculated average'.

MEASURES OF VARIATION

Range, average deviation and standard deviation

A normal distribution of data has a measure of central tendency, and a measure of variation within the distribution.

The simplest measure of variation is the *range,* or the difference between the largest and smallest item in the distribution. The symbol for range is *R.* For the patients' temperature distribution previously cited, $R = 0.7°C$ (37.3°C to 38.0°C).

However, the amount by which a given single item in a set of values differs from the mean of those values is the *deviation.* A deviation is considered positive if the item is larger than the mean and negative if it is smaller. One of the measures used to describe how much, on average, an item deviates from the mean is called the *average deviation.* It results from summing all the absolute deviations from the mean without regard to algebraic sign and dividing by the number of deviations. The formula for average deviation (AD) is:

$$\text{Average deviation} = \frac{\text{sum of absolute deviations}}{\text{number of deviations}} = \frac{\Sigma(\bar{X} - X)}{n} = \frac{\Sigma d}{n}$$

Example 16.1

The diameter of a sample of a nylon suture material at different points on the strand was found to be 0.125 mm, 0.132 mm, 0.112 mm, 0.120 mm, 0.125 mm, 0.120 mm, 0.130 mm, 0.117 mm, 0.112 mm and 0.135 mm. Calculate the mean and the average deviation.

The data is tabulated, the mean calculated, then the absolute deviation from the mean:

Diameter (mm)	Absolute deviation (mm)
0.125	0.002
0.132	0.009
0.112	0.011
0.120	0.003
0.125	0.002
0.120	0.003
0.130	0.007
0.117	0.006
0.112	0.011
0.135	0.012

$$\text{Mean} = \frac{1.228}{10} = 0.123 \text{ mm}$$

Absolute deviations are summed to calculate the average deviation:

$$\text{Average deviation} = \frac{0.066}{10} = 0.0066 \text{ or } 0.007 \text{ mm}$$

The more common measure of variation is the *standard deviation* of the items in a given set of data. Standard deviation is a measure of the accuracy of the mean and is obtained by: (i) squaring the deviations; (ii) summing the squared deviations; (iii) dividing by the number of deviations minus 1; (iv) calculating the square root of the quotient of the division. The formula for standard deviation (abbreviated to σ, S.D. or SD) is:

$$SD = \sqrt{\frac{(\text{Sum of deviations})^2}{\text{Number of deviations minus one}}} = \sqrt{\frac{\Sigma d^2}{n-1}}$$

(The $n-1$ in the formula is referred to as the 'degrees of freedom' or d.f.)

Example 16.2

The drug content of a sample of 500 mg capsules was assayed in a quality control procedure, and the following data were obtained: 508 mg, 493 mg, 518 mg, 509 mg, 484 mg, 511 mg, 500 mg, 489 mg, 504 mg and 496 mg. Calculate the mean and the standard deviation

Weight (mg)	Deviation (mg)	(Deviation)²
508	+ 7	49
493	− 8	64
518	+ 17	289
509	+ 8	64
484	− 17	289
511	+ 10	100
500	− 1	1
489	− 12	144
504	+ 3	9
496	− 5	25
5012		1034

$$\text{Mean} = \frac{5012}{10} = 501 \text{ mg}$$

$$\sigma = \sqrt{\frac{\Sigma d^2}{n-1}} = \sqrt{\frac{1034}{9}} = \sqrt{114.9} = 10.7 \text{ mg}$$

In order to determine the content-uniformity of solid dosage forms, the United States Pharmacopoeia employs a calculation termed *Relative Standard Deviation (RSD)* in which a test sample's standard deviation is divided by the mean, with the result expressed as a percentage. Thus, from the above example, the RSD would be:

$$RSD = \frac{SD}{Average} \times 100 = \frac{10.6}{501} \times 100 = 2.14\%.$$

The following approximate relationships may be used to compare the accuracy of measures of variation:

1. The average deviation is approximately $\frac{4}{5}$ of the standard deviation.
2. The range is never less than the standard deviation or more than seven times the standard deviation.

THE NORMAL DISTRIBUTION

For data that are normally distributed or symmetric, we can use parametric tests for evaluating the data if there is normality of variables. The data in a normal distribution curve lie within a symmetric frequency curve. To access the normal table, we standardize the observed value, X, to the standard normal deviate, z, by subtracting the mean, μ, from the observed value, x, and dividing the result by the standard deviation, σ:

$$\text{Standard normal deviate } (z) = \frac{X - \mu}{\sigma}$$

This enables removal of the units (e.g. kg or mg), and to use one normal table. Figure 16.1 shows the standard normal distribution (SND) interpreted in terms of a scale illustrating the number of standard deviations (σ) from the mean (μ). If the standard normal deviate (z) = 2, this means that the observation X is at a distance from the mean which equals 2 standard deviations. The normal distribution allows $z = \pm 3$ standard deviations. The mean of the unit normal distribution is equal to zero and its standard deviation is equal to 1. That is why the unit normal distribution is called $N(0,1)$ to differentiate it from the normal distribution in which mean μ and standard deviation σ is called $N(\mu,\sigma)$.

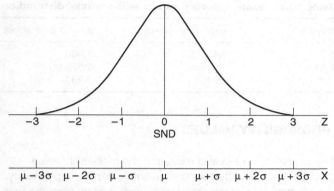

Fig. 16.1 Standard normal distribution (SND) interpreted in terms of a scale showing the number of standard deviations (σ) from the mean (μ).

SAMPLING VARIATION

The sample mean, x, and standard deviation, s, are used to estimate the population mean, μ, and the population standard deviation, σ, respectively. Different samples give different estimates for x. The difference between these sample means is due to sampling variation.

If we collect many independent samples of the same size, n, and calculate the sample mean of each, then frequency distribution of these means could be constructed. If n is large, the sampling distribution of the means tends to normal distribution with mean equal to the population mean. Approximately 95% of the sample means obtained by repeated sampling would lie within two standard errors above or below the population mean, μ (standard error = $\sigma/\sqrt{n}$). This fact can be used to construct a range of possible values of the unknown population mean, based on the observed sample mean and its standard error. Such a range is called a *confidence interval*.

Table 16.1 Some important values in the normal distribution

p value	z value (one-sided)	z value (two-sided)
0.05	1.645	1.960
0.01	2.325	2.575
0.001	3.090	3.290

PROBABILITY VALUES

The confidence interval is related to the probability value (p value) which is often used in scientific papers in pharmacy. If $z_{(\alpha)}$ is the value of the standard normal deviate from the unit normal table at level of significance equal to α, the term α is called the p value; p is the probability that the significance reached may be due to chance. If p is 5%, then the probability that the results may be due to chance (i.e. is not true, not genuine or not significant) is 5%. Thus, there is only a 95% confidence in the conclusion.

Some important values of the standard normal distribution are given in Table 16.1. To obtain significant results, the p value should be 0.05 or less. If the p value is greater than 0.05, then there are large amounts of error, and hence there is no significance.

STUDENT t-DISTRIBUTION

$t(\alpha, \text{d.f.} = n - 1)$: t stands for the Student t distribution which is an approximation for the unit normal distribution in cases where n is small or the standard deviation, σ, is unknown. The student t distribution has a mean of zero like the unit normal distribution but differs in allowing more spread or variation than the normal distribution. To access the t table requires the degrees of freedom and type I error, p. Figure 16.2 shows the normal distribution compared to t distribution with 5 degrees of freedom. The shape of the t distribution depends on the degrees of freedom. The fewer the degrees of freedom, the more spread out the t distribution becomes.

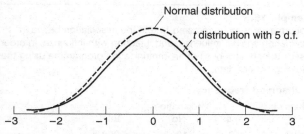

Fig. 16.2 The normal distribution compared to t distribution with 5 degrees of freedom.

The two-sided test is used when we do not know the direction of change in measurements either to the right or to the left, which is usually the condition in research. The one-sided test is used when it is known that the change will be in one direction, e.g. taking an antidiabetic medication, the outcome is to lower the blood glucose. However, it is best to undertake the two-sided test since it is conservative (i.e. more difficult to reach significance than using the one-sided test).

CHI SQUARED TEST

A different approach is required when dealing with qualitative data. When there are two qualitative variables, the data can be arranged in a contingency table. Categories for one variable define the rows, and categories for the other variable define the columns and observations are assigned to the appropriate cell of the contingency table. A contingency table is also used for discretized quantitative variables (continuous variables whose values have been grouped, e.g. when age is broken into groups).

A chi-squared (χ^2) test is used to test whether there is an association between the row variable and the column variable. It is a way of testing a hypothesis.

Example 16.3

A pharmacist may be required to test the association between vaccination against influenza, and infection with influenza, in order to assess the effectiveness of an immunization programme using the following sets of data:

(i) Observed frequency

Influenza	Vaccination		
	Yes	No	Total
Yes	40	160	200
No	440	280	720
Total	480	440	920

(ii) Expected frequency

Influenza	Vaccine	Placebo	Total
Yes	104.4	95.6	200
No	375.6	344.4	720
Total	480	440	920

The expected frequencies are calculated on the assumption that vaccination, and suffering from influenza are independent or not associated, i.e. we assume that the null hypothesis, H_0, is true and multiply the probabilities.

To test the hypothesis, follow these three steps:

1 Hypotheses

H_0: No association between influenza and vaccination.
H_A: Significant association between influenza and vaccination.

2 Test statistic

$$\chi^2 = \frac{(O_1 - E_1)^2}{E_1} + \frac{(O_2 - E_2)^2}{E_2} + \frac{(O_3 - E_3)^2}{E_3} + \frac{(O_4 - E_4)^2}{E_4}$$

where χ^2 is chi-squared notation, O is observed value and E is expected value.

$$\chi^2 = \frac{(40 - 104.4)^2}{104.4} + \frac{(160 - 95.6)^2}{95.6} + \frac{(440 - 375.6)^2}{375.6} + \frac{(280 - 344.4)^2}{344.4}$$

$$\chi^2 = 39.73 + 43.38 + 11.04 + 12.04 = 106.19$$

3 Conclusion

Compare χ^2 calculated with χ^2 table at degrees of freedom = (number of rows – l) × (number of columns – 1).

This gives $p < 0.001$, which indicates that there is significant association between infection with influenza and vaccination.

CORRELATION AND REGRESSION

Correlation measures the extent of relationship between two variables, while simple linear regression provides the prediction equation that quantifies such a relationship in the best way. Simple Pearson correlation and linear regression are two techniques used to investigate the linear association between two quantitative variables.

The correlation coefficient (r) has a value between -1 and $+1$, and equals zero if the two variables are not associated. It is positive if the two continuous X and Y variables have direct relation, i.e. they increase or decrease together. If the correlation coefficient is negative, the relationship is indirect, i.e. if X values increase, Y values decrease. The larger the value of r, the stronger is the association. The maximum value of 1 occurs in case of perfect correlation. In the case of perfect correlation, all the points lie exactly on a straight line. These relationships can be depicted further in scatter diagrams as shown in Figure 16.3A–E. Figure 16.3A shows that two variables X and Y are not associated and the relationship gives an r value of zero. Figure 16.3B shows two associated variables, which generally increase or decrease together giving an imperfect positive r value which is greater than 0 but less than 1. Figure 16.3C shows a perfect positive correlation, and r equals 1. Figure 16.3D shows an imperfect negative correlation where the r value is between zero and minus one. This shows that the two quantitative variables X and Y are associated inversely, such that as X increases, Y decreases; and as X decreases, Y increases. Finally, Figure 16.3E shows a perfect negative correlation, where the r value is equal to -1, and the association between the two variables is completely indirect. In this case, the two variables X and Y are associated indirectly, such that X increases when Y decreases, and X decreases when Y increases. However, a poor correlation may be statistically significant if the number of observations is very large, while a strong correlation may fail to achieve significance with only few observations.

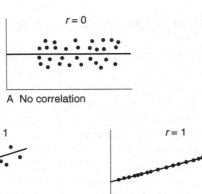

A No correlation

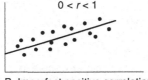

B Imperfect positive correlation

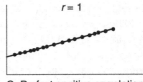

C Perfect positive correlation

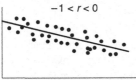

D Imperfect negative correlation

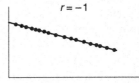

E Perfect negative correlation

Fig. 16.3 Scatter diagrams (A–E) showing different types of regression lines and corresponding values for their correlation coefficients.

STATISTICAL COMPUTATION USING STATISTICAL PACKAGES

Statistical analyses involve calculations using a wide variety of statistical formulae. Computers can perform all the operations that can be carried out on a calculator more quickly. On large sets of data, it can store all the steps of a calculation in a program. Operations can include storage, checking and sorting of data, and categorization of variables. Computation using a computer can be carried out in much wider terms than just calculation, and the extra features involved form a considerable part of many statistical analyses.

The process of statistical analysis could be divided into five stages. The first three stages (collecting, transferring and cleaning data) are often called data processing and the last two stages (organizing and calculating) are termed the statistical analysis.

Statistical analysis

Large sets of data may be analysed in several ways, but it is more efficient to go through a stage of organizing the data into a new data file before analysis. This new data file will contain categorized variables and derived variables from the recorded data, and it is usually more compact than the original one. The data might be reduced to a multi-way table which is then analysed. The process of applying statistical methods and formulae to data arranged for this purpose is termed statistical analysis. The task of producing graphs is also greatly eased by the availability of graphical software.

Statistical packages

To perform a particular method of statistical analysis on a computer, a program setting the statistical method is required. A set of programs integrated together into a single piece of software is called a package and such packages are the most convenient software to use for statistical analysis. For instance, packages such as *SPSS* (*Statistical Package for the Social Sciences*), *BMDP* (*BioMedical Data Processing*), *SAS* (*Statistical Analysis System*) and *STATA* (*Statistical Analysis*) are readily available. A spreadsheet is used to represent rows and columns of data. Basic arithmetic operations such as addition, subtraction, multiplication, division and exponentiation are performed on the data to give the statistical functions of sum, mean, standard deviation, and variance. Statistical analyses of data usually provide at least median, percentiles, confidence intervals, chi-square, *p* values and model fit. The analysed data may be displayed as bar and pie charts, histograms, error bars and box plots.

SELF-STUDY QUESTIONS

16.1 The systolic blood pressures (mm Hg) of 21 patients were recorded at a clinic:

127	132	129	138	134	128	123
128	136	127	122	127	129	126
140	121	130	128	126	122	127

Organize the data from the minimum to maximum values, and calculate the mean.
Find the median and the mode from the set of data.

16.2 The weights of a set of 11 capsules recorded in a quality control test were 300, 300, 315, 312, 294, 309, 303, 312, 306, 297 and 303 mg. Calculate the mean, the range, the average deviation and the standard deviation.

16.3 Fifteen samples of a potassium permanganate solution were assayed, and the results, in terms of percent (%) of potassium permanganate, were recorded:

2.52	2.46	2.42	2.61	2.52
2.44	2.52	2.60	2.57	2.48
2.47	2.50	2.51	2.55	2.43

Calculate the mean, and find the median and the mode for the recorded data.

16.4 During the production of penicillin tablets, a batch of 20 tablets were weighed individually and the following values (in mg) were obtained:

500	520	484	470	478
490	450	534	500	516
460	464	550	496	526
496	512	500	464	500

(a) Calculate the average weight of the tablets sampled.
(b) If the designated weight tolerance, based on average weight, is 7.5%, do all the tablets sampled fall within this limit?

16.5 The weights (in milligrams) of 20 tablets taken at random from a manufacturer's lot, were recorded:

104	96	98	101	100
99	102	103	100	97
102	100	102	98	99
101	101	100	97	99

Calculate the mean, the average deviation and the standard deviation for the recorded weights.

16.6 The average blood glucose of a sample of 100 normal adults is 100 mg/dL with standard deviation 5. What is the 95% confidence interval of the true blood glucose population mean (mg/dL)?

A 100 ± 0.5 **D** 100 ± 2.5

B 100 ± 1 **E** 100 ± 10

C 100 ± 1.5

For answers to these questions see page 294

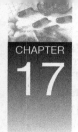

Introductory pharmacokinetics

After studying this chapter, you will be able to:

- **Understand the properties of first order kinetics and linear models**
- **Define, use, and calculate the parameters, k_{el}, $t_{1/2}$, V_d and AUC as they apply to a one compartment linear model**
- **Define, use and calculate clearance.**

INTRODUCTION TO PHARMACOKINETICS

Pharmacokinetics is the study of the kinetics of drug absorption, distribution and elimination. Each of these processes is associated with one or more pharmacokinetic parameters that determine the rate of the process. Pharmacokinetic principles have many applications in clinical services. It is feasible to determine the rate of drug absorption and elimination in order to characterize the concentration–time profile of a drug. Accurate methods are available for the estimation of drug levels in biological samples such as plasma, saliva, milk and urine. However, the measurement of drug concentration in the blood, serum or plasma is the most direct approach for assessing the pharmacokinetics of the drug in the body.

ONE COMPARTMENT IV BOLUS

Compartmental modelling is data-based modelling because the measured plasma concentration (C_p) after drug administration is used to choose the pharmacokinetic model.

The one compartment model assumes that the drug rapidly distributes in the body fluids when a drug is given by intravenous (IV) injection. According to this model the body is considered to behave as a single well-mixed container. The drug in the blood is in rapid equilibrium with drug in the extravascular tissues. The drug concentration may not be equal in each tissue or fluid, but it is assumed that they are proportional to the concentration of drug in the blood at all times. It is assumed that drug elimination follows first order kinetics. First order kinetics means that the rate of change of drug concentration by any process is directly proportional to the drug concentration remaining.

FIRST ORDER KINETICS

Elimination rate constant, k_{el}

For a linear model the rate of elimination (k_{el}) is constant, it does not change.

$$\text{Log } C_p = \frac{\log C_p^0 - k_{el}.t}{2.303}$$

where C_p is the plasma concentration at a given time, C_p^0 is the initial plasma concentration, k_{el} is the rate constant, and t is time (in minutes or hours).

The equation represents a straight line equation, of the form $y = a - b.t$ with a = intercept (log C_p^0) and b = slope ($-k_{el}$) and t is time. Thus, plotting log (C_p) versus (t) gives a straight line with a slope of ($-k_{el}$) and an intercept of log (C_p^0).

Half-life

Another property of first order kinetics is the half-life of elimination, $t_{1/2}$. The half-life is the time taken for the plasma concentration to fall to half its original value. Thus if C_p = concentration at the start and $C_p/2$ is the concentration one half-life later, then:

$$t_{1/2} = \frac{0.693}{k_{el}}$$

where $t_{1/2}$ is the half-life and k_{el} is elimination rate constant.

Example 17.1

Calculate the elimination rate constant for a drug that has an elimination half-life of 47 minutes, if it follows first order kinetics.

$$k_{el} = \frac{0.693}{t_{1/2}} = \frac{0.693}{47} = 0.0147 \text{ min}^{-1}$$

Example 17.2

After an intravenous bolus dose of 20 mg of a drug, blood samples were drawn from the patient and analysed at specific time intervals, giving the data shown in Table 17.1. What is the elimination half-life of the drug?

Figure 17.1 shows the plot of plasma drug level concentration ($\mu g/100$ mL) on the y-axis on a logarithmic scale, against time (h) on the x-axis on normal scale. From the plotted data, the straight line is extrapolated to time zero to determine the initial plasma drug concentration, which is found to be $80 \mu g/100$ mL. The time it takes to reduce that level to one-half, or $40 \mu g/100$ mL, is the elimination half-life. The $40 \mu g/100$ mL concentration intersects the straight line at 2.3 hours. Therefore, the elimination half-life is 2.3 hours. From Figure 17.1 it is possible to determine the percentages of drug eliminated at multiples of half-lives:

$C_p \to C_p/2$ in 1 half-life, i.e. 50.0% eliminated 50.0%
$C_p \to C_p/4$ in 2 half-lives, i.e. 25.0% eliminated 75.0%
$C_p \to C_p/8$ in 3 half-lives, i.e. 12.5% eliminated 87.5%
$C_p \to C_p/16$ in 4 half-lives, i.e. 6.25% eliminated 93.75%

Table 17.1   Concentration versus time data

Time (h)	C_p ($\mu g/100$ mL)
1	63.1
2	43.5
3	34.7
4	24.2
6	13.7
8	6.8
10	3.8
12	2.0

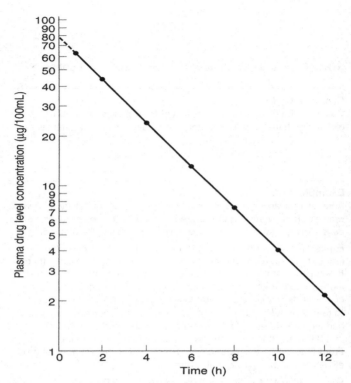

Fig. 17.1 Plasma drug level concentration (µg/100 mL) against time (h)

$C_p \rightarrow C_p/32$ in 5 half-lives, i.e. 3.125% eliminated 96.875%
$C_p \rightarrow C_p/64$ in 6 half-lives, i.e. 1.563% eliminated 98.438%
$C_p \rightarrow C_p/128$ in 7 half-lives, i.e. 0.781% eliminated 99.219%

Thus over 99% is eliminated in 7 half-lives.

Apparent volume of distribution, V_d

From the previous equation: $\log C_p = \log C_p^0 - k_{el}.t/2.303$, we can calculate the plasma concentration at any time (C_p) when we know k_{el} and C_p^0. However, we may not know C_p^0 ahead of time, but we do know the dose in mass units, e.g. in mg.

To calculate C_p^0 we need to know the volume that the drug is distributed into, i.e. the apparent volume of the mixing container, the body. This apparent volume of distribution (V_d) is not a physiological volume; it is a mathematical factor relating the amount of drug in the body and the concentration of drug in the measured compartment, usually plasma.
After an intravenous dose of a drug is administered, the initial amount of drug in the body is the dose. Thus:

$$V_d = \frac{Dose}{C_p^0}$$

where V_d is the apparent volume of distribution (in litres), dose is the amount of drug (mg) given, and C_p^0 is the initial plasma concentration (usually in micrograms per mL).

Example 17.3
A patient received a single intravenous dose of 100 mg of a medication that produced an immediate blood concentration of 2.7 micrograms of medication per millilitre. Calculate the apparent volume of distribution.

$$V_d = \frac{Dose}{C_p^0} = \frac{100 \text{ mg}}{2.7 \text{ µg/mL}} = \frac{100 \text{ mg}}{2.7 \text{ mg/L}} = 37 \text{ L}$$

Area under the plasma concentration–time curve, AUC

Example 17.4
After an IV bolus dose of 300 mg of a drug, the data in Table 17.2 were collected. The data were plotted as shown in Figure 17.2.

Table 17.2 Concentration versus time data

Time (h)	C_p (µg/mL)
1	70
2	52
3	36
4	25
6	12
8	7
10	5

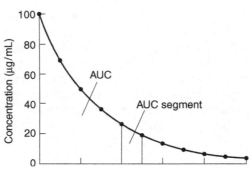

Fig. 17.2 Linear plot of concentration versus time showing AUC and AUC segment

Note that Figure 17.2 is a linear plot and it shows that the total area under the curve is the AUC. The AUC is calculated by adding all the AUC segments together. Each very narrow segment has an area = $C_p.dt$. Thus the total area is given by the equation:

$$AUC = \frac{Dose}{k_{el}.V_d} = \frac{C_p^0}{k_{el}}$$

ESTIMATION OF CREATININE CLEARANCE RATE (CL_{CR})

The kidneys receive about 20% of the cardiac output (blood flow) and filter approximately 125 mL per minute of plasma. When the kidney function is reduced, the quantity of plasma filtered per minute decreases, with an accompanying decrease in drug clearance. Drug elimination by the kidneys can often be correlated with blood urea nitrogen (BUN), serum creatinine (Sr_{Cr}) and creatinine clearance (CL_{Cr}). The BUN and Sr_{Cr} are less useful indices of renal function than the CL_{Cr} because they are influenced by other factors such as state of hydration and age. Creatinine, which is a breakdown product of muscle metabolism, is generally produced at a constant rate in the body. Since creatinine is eliminated from the body essentially through renal filtration, poor kidney performance results in a reduced creatinine clearance rate. The normal adult value of serum creatinine is 0.7–1.5 mg/dL. However, as patients age, both the production and clearance of creatinine decreases. Therefore, an elderly patient with a normal serum creatinine of 1 mg/dL may have a CL_{Cr} of much less than 100 mL/min (normal CL_{Cr} is 100–120 mL/min for a 70 kg adult). The creatinine clearance rate represents the volume of blood plasma that is cleared of creatinine by kidney filtration per minute (units are mL/min). The filtration rate of the kidney can therefore be estimated by the creatinine clearance rate (CL_{Cr}) through the use of empiric formulae based on the patient's age, weight and serum creatinine value. The Jelliffe, and Cockcroft–Gault equations are two methods commonly used to calculate CL_{Cr} as shown below. For females, the calculated CL_{Cr} values are reduced.

By the Jelliffe equation

For males:

$$\text{Creatinine clearance rate } (CL_{Cr}) = \frac{98 - 0.8 \times (\text{patient's age in years} - 20)}{\text{serum creatinine in mg/dL}}$$

For females:

$CL_{Cr} = 0.9 \times CL_{Cr}$ determined using formula for males.

By the Cockcroft–Gault equation

For males:

$$CL_{Cr} = \frac{(140 - \text{patient's age in years}) \times \text{body weight in kg}}{72 \times \text{serum creatinine in mg/dL}}$$

For females:

$CL_{Cr} = 0.85 \times CL_{Cr}$ determined using formula for males.

Example 17.4

Determine the creatinine clearance rate for a 60-year-old male patient weighing 70 kg and having a serum creatinine of 2 mg/dL. Use both the Jelliffe, and Cockcroft–Gault equations.

By the Jelliffe equation:

$$CL_{Cr} = \frac{98 - 0.8 \times (60 - 20)}{2(\text{mg/dL})} = \frac{98 - (0.8 \times 40)}{2 \text{ (mg/dL)}} = \frac{98 - 32}{2} = \frac{66}{2} = 33 \text{ mL/min}$$

By the Cockcroft–Gault equation:

$$CL_{Cr} = \frac{(140 - 60) \times 70}{72 \times 2 \text{ (mg/dL)}} = \frac{80 \times 70}{144} = \frac{5600}{144} = 38.9 \text{ mL/min}$$

There are many situations in clinical pharmacokinetics that do not fit the one compartment model discussed in this chapter. A more specialized textbook is required for these more complex situations.

SELF-STUDY QUESTIONS

17.1 A patient received a single intravenous dose of 5 mg of diazepam. A blood sample was drawn and it contained 22 µg/100 mL. Calculate the apparent volume of distribution for the drug.

17.2 Calculate the elimination rate constant for a drug having an elimination half-life of 3.5 hours. Assume that first-order kinetics occurs.

17.3 What percentage of an originally administered intravenous dose of a drug remains in the body following five half-lives? Assume first-order pharmacokinetics.

17.4 If 500 mg of a drug are administered intravenously and the resultant drug plasma concentration is determined to be 14.3 µg/mL, calculate the apparent volume of distribution.

17.5 The volume of distribution for chlordiazepoxide has been determined to be 28 litres. Calculate the expected drug plasma concentration of the drug, in micrograms per decilitre, immediately after an intravenous dose of 10 mg.

17.6 A calculated pharmacokinetic parameter that gives an estimate of the renal function of a patient is the:

(a) blood urea nitrogen
(b) creatinine clearance
(c) free water clearance
(d) serum creatinine
(e) urine creatinine

17.7 Assuming complete absorption and an elimination half-life of 6 hours, how many mg of a drug will remain in the body 18 hours after administering a 500 mg dose? Assume linear pharmacokinetics (i.e. first order):

(a) 12.5   **(c)** 62.5   **(e)** 300
(b) 25.0   **(d)** 125

17.8 Determine the half-life of a drug if it appears to be eliminated from the body at a rate constant of 25% per hour. (Assume that first-order kinetics occur):

(a) <1 hour   **(c)** 5.6 hours   **(e)** >10 hours
(b) 2.8 hours   **(d)** 8.0 hours

17.9 Estimate the plasma concentration of a drug when 100 mg is given by IV bolus to a 154-lb patient if her volume of distribution is 1.2 L/kg:

(a) 0.50 mg/L   **(c)** 3.00 mg/L   **(e)** 58.33 mg/L
(b) 1.19 mg/L   **(d)** 7.50 mg/L

For answers to these questions see page 295

18 Mock registration examination paper

The Open Book paper includes 20 calculation questions. The RPSGB has on their website sample papers which give 10 practice calculation questions. There follows a mock 20-question test paper. It is difficult to give guidance on timing, but it is worth noting that most examinees agree that time is very short in the examination. Therefore, spending a long time on the calculations will reduce the time remaining for the rest of the paper. You will need to have access to a copy of the BNF in order to complete this paper.

INSTRUCTIONS

1. For each question there are five options, A, B, C, D and E. Choose only one of the options as your answer for each question.
2. You should answer the questions as though you were a registered pharmacist, not a preregistration trainee.
3. You will score one mark for each correct answer: no marks will be deducted for incorrect answers or omissions.
4. The use of calculators is not permitted.

1 The following is an extract from a prescription:

Prednisolone 5 mg tablets Take 25 mg daily for 4 days then reduce by 5 mg every 4 days until the course is finished (Total course 20 days)

Which one of the following is the exact number of prednisolone 5 mg tablets that you should supply?

A 100
B 80
C 60
D 40
E 20

2 Ranitidine tablets are available as tablets containing ranitidine hydrochloride equivalent to 150 mg and 300 mg of ranitidine. To prepare ranitidine 150 mg tablets, what weight of ranitidine hydrochloride is needed in each tablet? (Molecular weights: Ranitidine: $C_{13}H_{22}N_4O_3S$ = 314.4; Ranitidine hydrochloride: $C_{13}H_{22}N_4O_3S.HCl$ = 350.9):

A 134 mg
B 150 mg
C 167 mg
D 269 mg
E 335 mg

3 You receive a prescription for enalapril maleate 1.25 mg qds for 30 days. The lowest strength preparation of enalapril maleate available to you is 2.5 mg tablets, each weighing 80 mg. After discussion with the prescriber, you decide to supply 200 mg powders each containing 1.25 mg of enalapril maleate using lactose as a diluent. What weight of lactose needs to be added to the crushed tablets to supply the exact amount required on the prescription?

A 4.8 g
B 9.6 g
C 14.4 g
D 19.2 g
E 24.4 g

4 A tablet contains 4% w/w of binder, which is added to the other ingredients during granulation as a 20% w/v solution. What volume of this solution is required for the manufacture of 500 000 × 100 mg tablets?

A 100 L
B 10 L
C 4 L
D 2 L
E 0.4 L

5 Approximately how many millimoles of sodium ions are there in 60 mL of sodium bicarbonate solution 1.26%? (Atomic weights: hydrogen = 1, carbon = 12, oxygen = 16, sodium = 23)

A 0.4 mmol **C** 4 mmol **E** 90 mmol
B 0.9 mmol **D** 9 mmol

6 A boy weighing 20 kg has been admitted to hospital for surgery. During the operation he is given an intravenous dose of 3 micrograms/kg fentanyl injection. The fentanyl injection contains 50 micrograms/mL. What volume of fentanyl injection should he have been given?

A 0.06 mL **C** 0.6 mL **E** 1.2 mL
B 0.4 mL **D** 0.8 mL

7 Mr D has cardiovascular disease and is taking Peptac® suspension, 20 mL tds pc. You are asked to calculate how many mmol of sodium ions Mr D receives each day from the Peptac® suspension. Which one of the following is correct?

A 3.1 mmol **C** 12.4 mmol **E** 186.0 mmol
B 9.3 mmol **D** 37.2 mmol

8 This question concerns the following formula that can be used to calculate paediatric doses:

$$\text{Approximate dose for child} = \frac{\text{surface area of patient (m}^2)}{1.8} \times \text{adult dose}$$

If the adult dose of a medicine is 200 mg, what is the approximate dose for a 5 year old with a body surface area of 0.65 m²?

A 1.8 mg **C** 62 mg **E** 111 mg
B 47 mg **D** 72 mg

9 What volume of alcohol 95% v/v is needed to produce 2.5 litres of 73% v/v?

A 3.25 L **C** 1.92 L **E** 0.31 L
B 2.77 L **D** 0.52 L

10 While visiting a ward you are asked to calculate the volume of Potassium Chloride Concentrate 15% w/v that should be added to a 500 mL bag of sodium chloride 0.9% w/v infusion to produce a concentration of 10 mmol potassium ions per litre. The volume of Potassium Chloride Concentrate required is:

A	2.5 mL	**C**	5.0 mL	**E**	10.0 mL
B	4.0 mL	**D**	7.5 mL		

11 A patient requests 250 g of 0.5% w/w salicylic acid in Hydrous Ointment BP. What weight of salicylic acid would be required to prepare this for the patient?

A	1.25 g	**C**	50 g	**E**	125 g
B	12.5 g	**D**	75 g		

12 A patient has been prescribed dopexamine hydrochloride by intravenous infusion, 500 nanograms/kg/min. You ascertain that the patient weighs 72 kg. Using a 400 micrograms/mL infusion solution, what volume per minute should the infusion be set at?

A	0.09 mL	**C**	1.1 mL	**E**	11.1 mL
B	0.9 mL	**D**	9.0 mL		

Questions 13 and 14 concern the following weights of proflavine hemisulphate powder:

A	0.02 g	**C**	2.0 g	**E**	200 g
B	0.2 g	**D**	20 g		

Select from A to E which one of the above is the correct weight required to prepare:

13 400 mL of a 1 in 2000 solution of proflavine hemisulphate

14 8 litres of a 0.025% solution of proflavine hemisulphate

Questions 15 and 16 concern the following quantities:

A   30 g   C   5 g   E   2.5 g
B   25 g   D   3 g

Select from A to E which one of the above is correct:

15 The weight of erythromycin contained in 30 mL of
500 mg/5 mL elixir

16 The weight of glucose contained in 500 mL of 5%
infusion

17 The following question consists of a statement in the
left-hand column followed by a second statement in the
right-hand column. Decide whether the first statement is true
or false. Decide whether the second statement is true or false.
Then choose:

A   If both statements are true and the second statement is a
    correct explanation of the first statement
B   If both statements are true but the second statement is
    NOT a correct explanation of the first statement
C   If the first statement is true but the second statement is
    false
D   If the first statement is false but the second statement is
    true
E   If both statements are false

Concerns the following scenario:
You receive a telephone call from a junior doctor working in
the hospital's accident and emergency department. He is
treating a patient with ventricular arrhythmias following
myocardial infarction, and has already given him 150 mg
mexiletine hydrochloride as a bolus dose. He now wants to
start an infusion of mexiletine hydrochloride using a 0.1%
solution and asks you to advise on the infusion rate.

First statement	Second statement
The infusion rate should be set at 10 mL/min for the first 60 minutes	The initial infusion rate of mexiletine hydrochloride for the treatment of ventricular arrhythmias is 250 mg as a 0.1% solution for the first 60 minutes

Directions for questions 18, 19 and 20. The remaining questions are followed by three responses. ONE or MORE of the responses is (are) correct. Decide which of the responses is (are) correct. Then choose:

A If (i), (ii) and (iii) are correct
B If (i) and (ii) only are correct
C If (ii) and (iii) only are correct
D If (i) only is correct
E If (iii) only is correct

18 Which of the following will provide a 0.2 mg dose of adrenaline (epinephrine)?

(i) 2 mL of a 100 microgram/mL solution
(ii) 0.2 mL of a 0.1% w/v solution
(iii) 0.02 mL of a 1 in 10 000 solution

19 A 6-year-old patient weighing 20 kg has been prescribed pethidine by intramuscular injection for pain. Which of the following doses is/are within BNF recommended limits?

(i) 0.8 mL of the 50 mg/mL injection
(ii) 1.2 mL of the 50 mg/mL injection
(iii) 1.5 mL of the 50 mg/mL injection

Question 20 concerns the following extracts from a prescription and a formula sheet:

Prescription

Levothyroxine Suspension

50 micrograms in 5 mL

Supply 40 mL

45 micrograms to be taken daily

Formula for Levothyroxine Suspension

Levothyroxine tablets (50 micrograms)	q.s.
Compound Tragacanth Powder BP	1 g
Syrup BP	20 mL
Concentrated Chloroform Water BPC	2.5 mL
Purified Water to	100 mL

20 Which of the following is/are true?

(i) To dispense the quantity prescribed above, the formula should contain 0.8 mL of Concentrated Chloroform Water BPC

(ii) The child should be given 4.5 mL each day

(iii) To dispense the quantity prescribed above, the formula should contain 8 × 50 micrograms levothyroxine tablets

For answers to these questions see page 295

CHAPTER 1

1.1	0.6	**1.21**	1.58	**1.41**	74.922
1.2	0.6	**1.22**	0.15	**1.42**	1.373
1.3	3.6	**1.23**	0.45	**1.43**	9.012
1.4	12.8	**1.24**	0.01	**1.44**	132.905
1.5	7.5	**1.25**	1.08	**1.45**	4.008
1.6	0.1	**1.26**	24.65	**1.46**	58.933
1.7	1.0	**1.27**	0.13	**1.47**	196.967
1.8	1.9	**1.28**	0.08	**1.48**	138.906
1.9	17.6	**1.29**	1.80	**1.49**	1.008
1.10	30.0	**1.30**	0.53	**1.50**	231.036
1.11	4.37	**1.31**	26.982	**1.51**	39.95
1.12	2.72	**1.32**	121.76	**1.52**	209.0
1.13	0.319	**1.33**	10.812	**1.53**	79.90
1.14	24.3	**1.34**	1210 100	**1.54**	3.545
1.15	105 000	**1.35**	0.63546	**1.55**	19.00
1.16	1370	**1.36**	1.6493	**1.56**	4.003
1.17	823	**1.37**	12 690	**1.57**	1.750
1.18	7.84	**1.38**	309.74	**1.58**	16.00
1.19	5010	**1.39**	3.9098	**1.59**	22.99
1.20	259	**1.40**	1.4091	**1.60**	0.4787

CHAPTER 2

2.1	**(a)** 1.296 g	**(e)** 56.83 mL	**(i)** 4546.4 mL
	(b) 1.944 g	**(f)** 284.13 mL	**(j)** 3.55 mL
	(c) 10.37 g	**(g)** 28.41 mL	**(k)** 972 mg
	(d) 25.92 g	**(h)** 1136.6 mL	**(l)** 3.888 g

	(m)	21.38 g	(q)	7.10 mL	(u)	198.89 mL
	(n)	4.212 g	(r)	2.916 g	(v)	29.81 g
	(o)	1704.9 mL	(s)	5.184 g	(w)	0.89 mL
	(p)	9.396 g	(t)	23.98 g		
2.2	(a)	165.4 g	(d)	352.8 mg	(g)	248.3 mg
	(b)	180.2 mg	(e)	352.3 mg	(h)	781.8 g
	(c)	441.4 g	(f)	494.0 mg	(i)	504.1 mg
2.3	(a)	1564 g	(e)	4563 g	(i)	16.54 g
	(b)	1.652 g	(f)	3.608 g	(j)	908.4 g
	(c)	1262 g	(g)	27.33 g	(k)	1.191 g
	(d)	4.244 g	(h)	889.2 g		
2.4	(a)	19.70 g	(d)	7.118 g	(g)	9.618 g
	(b)	5.367 g	(e)	2.713 g		
	(c)	4.165 g	(f)	7.809 g		
2.5	(a)	23.67 mmol	(d)	31.19 mmol	(g)	13.45 mmol
	(b)	19.21 mmol	(e)	13.65 mmol	(h)	12.30 mmol
	(c)	16.65 mmol	(f)	19.59 mmol	(i)	6.659 mmol
2.6	(a)	14.01 g	(e)	72.93 g	(i)	371.6 mg
	(b)	686.5 mg	(f)	261.6 g	(j)	223.4 g
	(c)	22.99 mg	(g)	80.16 mg		
	(d)	1.951 g	(h)	3.046 g		
2.7	(a)	84.01 mg	(c)	267.5 mg	(e)	51.70 mg
	(b)	233.8 mg	(d)	252.0 mg	(f)	103.4 mg
2.8	(a)	0.30 mEq	(c)	0.53 mEq	(e)	0.52 mEq
	(b)	0.60 mEq	(d)	1.58 mEq	(f)	0.87 mEq
2.9	(a)	22.68 kg	(e)	58.97 kg	(i)	28.58 kg
	(b)	13.61 kg	(f)	3.538 kg	(j)	58.06 kg
	(c)	99.79 kg	(g)	54.43 kg		
	(d)	88.45 kg	(h)	96.62 kg		

2.10 (a) 209.44 pounds   (e) 92.59 pounds
         (b) 176.37 pounds   (f) 1.10 pounds
         (c) 46.30 pounds   (g) 156.53 pounds
         (d) 3.31 pounds

2.11 (a) 88.90 cm   (c) 48.26 cm   (e) 96.52 cm
         (b) 27.94 cm   (d) 68.58 cm   (f) 68.58 cm

2.12 (a) 1.270 m   (c) 1.753 m
         (b) 1.854 m   (d) 1.397 m

2.13 (a) 20.47 inches   (f) 36.61 inches
         (b) 32.28 inches   (g) 29.53 inches
         (c) 11.81 inches   (h) 74.80 inches
         (d) 59.06 inches   (i) 57.48 inches
         (e) 82.68 inches   (j) 80.71 inches

2.14 (a) 39.2°F   (e) 86.0°F   (i) 102.6°F
         (b) −4.0°F   (f) 44.6°F   (j) 77.0°F
         (c) 33.8°F   (g) 98.6°F
         (d) 59.0°F   (h) 68.0°F

2.15 (a) 36.7°C   (e) 0°C   (i) 4.4°C
         (b) 40.0°C   (f) −23.3°C   (j) −56.7°C
         (c) 65.6°C   (g) 11.1°C
         (d) 48.9°C   (h) 25.6°C

CHAPTER 3

3.1 (a) 4.0% v/v   (j) 0.082% w/v   (s) 0.0055%
        (b) 1.0% v/v   (k) 0.19% w/v   (t) 1.2% v/v
        (c) 0.45% w/v   (l) 0.075%   (u) 0.042% w/v
        (d) 0.30% w/v   (m) 15% v/v   (v) 0.087%
        (e) 0.00040%   (n) 1.4% w/v   (w) 1.0% v/v
        (f) 0.0025%   (o) 0.055% w/v   (x) 0.011% w/v
        (g) 0.11% w/v   (p) 13% v/v   (y) 0.14% w/v
        (h) 0.056% w/v   (q) 0.36%
        (i) 12% v/v   (r) 0.32% w/v

3.2	(a) 1.00 g	(d) 0.73 g	(g) 0.25 g
	(b) 1.33 g	(e) 1.20 g	(h) 1.29 g
	(c) 5.71 g	(f) 1.33 g	(i) 3.33 g

3.3	(a) 1 in 4000	(d) 1 in 40 000	(g) 1 in 1250
	(b) 1 in 2222	(e) 1 in 22 222	
	(c) 1 in 1818	(f) 1 in 1429	

3.4	(a)	Hard paraffin	24.14% w/w
		Soft paraffin	48.28% w/w
		Liquid paraffin	27.59% w/w
	(b)	Hard paraffin	13.33% w/w
		Soft paraffin	66.67% w/w
		Liquid paraffin	20.00% w/w
	(c)	Hard paraffin	12.12% w/w
		Soft paraffin	66.67% w/w
		Liquid paraffin	21.21% w/w
	(d)	Hard paraffin	17.24% w/w
		Soft paraffin	68.97% w/w
		Liquid paraffin	13.79% w/w
	(e)	Hard paraffin	16.13% w/w
		Soft paraffin	70.97% w/w
		Liquid paraffin	12.90% w/w
	(f)	Hard paraffin	19.35% w/w
		Soft paraffin	58.06% w/w
		Liquid paraffin	22.58% w/w

3.5	(a) 1.5 mg/mL	(e) 8 mg/mL	(i) 22 mg/mL
	(b) 2.5 mg/mL	(f) 9 mg/mL	(j) 26 mg/mL
	(c) 4 mg/mL	(g) 12 mg/mL	
	(d) 6.5 mg/mL	(h) 18 mg/mL	

3.6	(a) 0.20 g	(e) 0.63 g	(i) 0.84 g
	(b) 0.03 g	(f) 1.20 g	(j) 2.40 g
	(c) 0.13 g	(g) 3.12 g	(k) 1.17 g
	(d) 1.60 g	(h) 2.10 g	

3.7

(a)	0.08% w/v	**(m)**	6.4% w/v
(b)	0.12% w/v	**(n)**	0.034% w/v
(c)	5.0% w/v	**(o)**	1.8% w/w
(d)	0.58% w/v	**(p)**	19% w/v
(e)	0.25% w/v	**(q)**	2.6% w/v
(f)	0.0020% w/v	**(r)**	0.050% w/w
(g)	0.17% w/w	**(s)**	4.0% w/v
(h)	0.0075% w/w	**(t)**	0.22% w/v
(i)	1.5% w/v	**(u)**	7.2% w/v
(j)	0.17% w/w	**(v)**	32% w/v
(k)	0.30% w/v	**(w)**	2.5% w/w
(l)	0.60% w/w		

3.8

(a)	200 mg	**(e)**	450 mg	**(i)**	200 mg
(b)	297 mg	**(f)**	150 mg	**(j)**	204 mg
(c)	306 mg	**(g)**	765 mg		
(d)	450 mg	**(h)**	150 mg		

3.9

(a)
Resorcinol	5% w/w
Precipitated sulphur	10% w/w
Zinc oxide	40% w/w
Emulsifying ointment	45% w/w

(b)
Calamine	7% w/w
Arachis oil	30% w/w
Emulsifying wax	6% w/w
Water	to 100% w/w

(c)
Starch	35% w/w
Zinc oxide	40% w/w
Olive oil	10% w/w
Wool fat	15% w/w

(d)
Chlorhexidine gluconate 20% solution	5% w/w
Cetomacrogol emulsifying wax	25% w/w
Liquid paraffin	10% w/w
Water	60% w/w

(e)
Wool fat	5% w/w
Hard paraffin	2.5% w/w
Cetostearyl alcohol	7.5% w/w
Soft paraffin	85% w/w

(f)	Ichthammol		5% w/w
	Cetostearyl alcohol		3% w/w
	Wool fat		10% w/w
	Zinc cream		to 100% w/w

3.10
- **(a)** 0.50% w/w
- **(b)** 0.19% w/v
- **(c)** 0.66%
- **(d)** 0.60% w/v
- **(e)** 1.43% v/v
- **(f)** 0.28% w/v
- **(g)** 2.80% w/v
- **(h)** 0.10%
- **(i)** 0.14% w/v
- **(j)** 0.36% w/v
- **(k)** 0.15% w/w
- **(l)** 0.22% w/v
- **(m)** 4.4% w/v
- **(n)** 0.97% v/v
- **(o)** 0.67% w/v
- **(p)** 0.67% v/v
- **(q)** 1.50% w/w

3.11
- **(a)** 2.20 g, 1.10 mL
- **(b)** 5.00 g, 2.50 mL
- **(c)** 14.32 g, 7.16 mL
- **(d)** 3.23 g, 1.62 mL
- **(e)** 3.88 g, 1.94 mL
- **(f)** 7.21 g, 3.60 mL
- **(g)** 7.34 g, 3.67 mL
- **(h)** 6.61 g, 3.31 mL
- **(i)** 12.76 g, 6.38 mL

3.12
- **(a)** 0.75% w/v
- **(b)** 1.07% w/v
- **(c)** 0.84% w/v
- **(d)** 0.14% w/v
- **(e)** 3.55% w/v
- **(f)** 1.03% w/v

3.13
- **(a)** 3.42 mEq
- **(b)** 0.77 mEq
- **(c)** 1.79 mEq
- **(d)** 0.81 mEq
- **(e)** 2.10 mEq

CHAPTER 4

4.1 **(a)** 55.0 µg **(b)** 83.4 µg

4.2 1.68 mg

4.3 **(a)** 412 mg **(b)** 341 mg **(c)** 311 mg

4.4 2.19 g

4.5 551 µg

4.6	**(a)** 368 mg	**(b)** 484 mg	**(c)** 409 mg

4.7   2.73 mg

4.8	**(a)** 270 mg	**(b)** 332 mg

4.9   5.62 mg

4.10   5.36 mg

4.11	**(a)** 2.29 mg	**(b)** 2.32 mg	**(c)** 2.19 mg

4.12	**(a)** 664 μg	**(b)** 633 μg

4.13	**(a)** 27.9 mg	**(b)** 33.6 mg	**(c)** 30.8 mg

4.14	**(a)** 39.9 μg	**(b)** 48.2 μg

4.15	**(a)** 5.35 mg/5 mL	**(b)** 4.98 mg/5 mL

4.16	**(a)** 347 mg	**(b)** 294 mg

4.17   7.32 mg

4.18	**(a)** 61.0 mg/mL	**(b)** 56.1 mg/mL

4.19   No: 12.4 mg of dinitrate is equivalent to 10 mg mono-nitrate

4.20   6.08 mg

4.21	**(a)** 21.5 mg	**(d)** 5.05 mg	**(g)** 56.6 mg
	(b) 1.81 mg	**(e)** 0.871 mg	**(h)** 38.4 mg
	(c) 32.5 mg	**(f)** 5.88 g	**(i)** 31.8 μg

4.22	**(a)** 65.7 mg	**(b)** 23.2 mg	**(c)** 65.0 mg

4.23 **(a)** 169 mg   **(c)** 122 mg   **(e)** 122 mg
          (b) 122 mg   **(d)** 136 mg   **(f)** 148 mg

4.24 **(a)** Strength   28.0 mg/100 mL
          Single dose   4.20 mg
          Volume of dose   15.0 mL

          (b) Strength   26.3 mg/100 mL
          Single dose   3.95 mg
          Volume of dose   15.0 mL

          (c) Strength   26.6 mg/100 mL
          Single dose   3.99 mg
          Volume of dose   15.0 mL

          (d) Strength   27.2 mg/100 mL
          Single dose   4.7 mg
          Volume of dose   15.0 mL

CHAPTER 5

5.1	1.17 g	**5.5**	4.62 g	**5.9**	8.6 mL
5.2	0.89 g	**5.6**	31.11 g	**5.10**	1.5 mL
5.3	63.94 g	**5.7**	26.2 mL	**5.11**	42.3 mL
5.4	17.92 g	**5.8**	21.3 mL		

5.12 6 g is required, which is 6.3 mL

5.13 6.25 mL is required, which is 7.22 g

5.14 50 g is required, which is 54.3 mL

5.15 10 g is required, which is 8.4 mL

5.16 3.75 mL is required, which is 4.50 g

5.17 The syrup has a density of 1.362 g/mL, so it does not comply

5.18 It should weigh between 328.75 g and 333.25 g

5.19 The lemon syrup has a density of 1.271 g/mL, so it is too low

5.20 The syrup has a density of 1.326 g/mL, so it complies

CHAPTER 6

6.1	**(a)** 3.33%	**(d)** 1.39%	**(g)** 100.00%			
	(b) 333.33%	**(e)** 25.00%				
	(c) 0.20%	**(f)** 1.67%				

6.2	**(a)** 24 mL	**(e)** 7 mL	**(i)** 7 mL
	(b) 2 mL	**(f)** 100 mL	**(j)** 0.1 mL
	(c) 10 mL	**(g)** 10 mL	
	(d) 2.4 mL	**(h)** 6 mL	

6.3	**(a)** 5 mL	**(e)** 1.5 L	**(i)** 1.05 mL
	(b) 1.35 mL	**(f)** 5 mL	**(j)** 1 mL
	(c) 2 mL	**(g)** 250 mL	
	(d) 12.5 mL	**(h)** 2 mL	

6.4	**(a)** 3.33 g	**(e)** 2.86 g	**(i)** 40.00 g
	(b) 8.70 g	**(f)** 6.67 g	**(j)** 10.00 g
	(c) 0.50 g	**(g)** 9.52 g	
	(d) 20.00 g	**(h)** 0.20 g	

6.5	**(a)** 167 mg No	**(f)** 20 g Yes	
	(b) 2.5 g Yes	**(g)** 83 mg No	
	(c) 200 mg Just	**(h)** 200 mg Just	
	(d) 25 mg No	**(i)** 833 mg Yes	
	(e) 28.57 g Yes		

6.6   **(a)** 4.00%   **(d)** 12.50%   **(g)** 2.00%
     (b) 0.12%   **(e)** 0.42%   **(h)** 4.76%
     (c) 142.86%   **(f)** 37.04%

6.7   1 in 100

6.8   **(a)** Yes   **(d)** No   **(g)** No
     (b) Yes   **(e)** Yes
     (c) Yes   **(f)** Yes

6.9   **(a)** 15 mL   **(d)** 8 L   **(g)** 0.045 mL
     (b) 100 mL   **(e)** 12 mL   **(h)** 1.05 mL
     (c) 1.25 L   **(f)** 48 mL   **(i)** 60 mL

6.10 **(a)** 250 mg. Yes   **(c)** 500 mg. Yes
     (b) 20 mg. No   **(d)** 83 mg. No

6.11

(a) 110 mL
(b) 46 mL. This salt is the most soluble in water
(c) 1.62 L

CHAPTER 7

7.1
(a) Belladonna tincture   2 mL
Benzoic acid solution   1 mL
Glycerol   5 mL
Syrup   10 mL
Water   to 50 mL

(b) Belladonna tincture   4.8 mL
Benzoic acid solution   2.4 mL
Glycerol   12 mL
Syrup   24 mL
Water   to 120 mL

(c) Belladonna tincture   2.4 mL
Benzoic acid solution   1.2 mL

Glycerol	6 mL
Syrup	12 mL
Water	to 60 mL

7.2

(a)
Starch	10.5 g
Zinc oxide	9 g
Olive oil	6 g
Wool fat	4.5 g

(b)
Hydrocortisone	0.5 g
Oxytetracycline	1.5 g
Wool fat	5 g
White soft paraffin	43 g

(c)
White beeswax	1.5 g
Hard paraffin	2.25 g
Cetostearyl alcohol	3.75 g
Soft paraffin	67.5 g

(d)
Starch	10.5 g
Zinc oxide	9 g
Olive oil	6 g
Wool fat	4.5 g

(e)
Hydrocortisone	0.6 g
Oxytetracycline	1.8 g
Wool fat	6 g
White soft paraffin	51.6 g

(f)
Starch	26.25 g
Zinc oxide	22.5 g
Olive oil	15 g
Wool fat	11.25 g

(g)
Wool alcohols	3.6 g
Soft paraffin	6 g
Hard paraffin	14.4 g
Liquid paraffin	36 g

(h)
Hydrocortisone	0.3 g
Oxytetracycline	0.9 g
Wool fat	3 g
White soft paraffin	25.8 g

(i)

White beeswax	3 g
Hard paraffin	4.5 g
Cetostearyl alcohol	7.5 g
Soft paraffin	135 g

(j)

Wool alcohols	4.5 g
Soft paraffin	7.5 g
Hard paraffin	18 g
Liquid paraffin	45 g

7.3

(a)

Light magnesium carbonate	1.8 g
Sodium bicarbonate	3.0 g
Aromatic cardamom tincture	1.8 mL
Chloroform water, double strength	30 mL
Water	to 60 mL

(b)

Magnesium sulphate	60 g
Light magnesium carbonate	7.5 g
Concentrated peppermint water	3.75 g
Chloroform water, double strength	45 mL
Water	to 150 mL

(c)

Light magnesium carbonate	3.6 g
Sodium bicarbonate	6.0 g
Aromatic cardamom tincture	3.6 mL
Chloroform water, double strength	60 mL
Water	to 120 mL

(d)

Magnesium sulphate	30 g
Light magnesium carbonate	3.75 g
Concentrated peppermint water	1.875 g
Chloroform water, double strength	22.5 mL
Water	to 75 mL

(e)

Magnesium trisilicate	6 g
Light magnesium carbonate	9 g
Sodium bicarbonate	3 g
Chloroform water, double strength	60 mL
Water	to 120 mL

7.4

(a) Resorcinol — 1.5 g
Precipitated sulphur — 3 g
Zinc oxide — 12 g
Emulsifying ointment — 13.5 g

(b) Starch — 10.5 g
Zinc oxide — 12 g
Olive oil — 3 g
Wool fat — 4.5 g

(c) Wool fat — 3 g
Hard paraffin — 1.5 g
Cetostearyl alcohol — 4.5 g
Soft paraffin — 51 g

(d) Resorcinol — 6 g
Precipitated sulphur — 12 g
Zinc oxide — 48 g
Emulsifying ointment — 54 g

(e) Resorcinol — 1.5 g
Precipitated sulphur — 3 g
Zinc oxide — 12 g
Emulsifying ointment — 13.5 g

(f) Wool fat — 6 g
Hard paraffin — 3 g
Cetostearyl alcohol — 9 g
Soft paraffin — 102 g

(g) White beeswax — 1.2 g
Hard paraffin — 1.8 g
Cetostearyl alcohol — 3 g
Soft paraffin — 54 g

(h) Hard paraffin — 13.33 g
Soft paraffin — 70.0 g
Liquid paraffin — 16.67 g

(i) White beeswax — 2.4 g
Hard paraffin — 3.6 g
Cetostearyl alcohol — 6.0 g
Soft paraffin — 108 g

(j)	Ichthammol	3.0 g
	Cetostearyl alcohol	1.8 g
	Wool fat	6 g
	Zinc cream	to 60 g

7.5

(a)	Calamine	8.4 g
	Arachis oil	36 g
	Emulsifying wax	7.2 g
	Water	to 120 g
(b)	Chlorhexidine gluconate 20% solution	1.5 g
	Cetomacrogol emulsifying wax	7.5 g
	Liquid paraffin	3 g
	Water	to 30 g
(c)	Zinc oxide	18 g
	Arachis oil	21 g
	Wool fat	6 g
	Water	to 60 g
(d)	Calamine	10.5 g
	Arachis oil	45 g
	Emulsifying wax	9 g
	Water	to 150 g
(e)	Chlorhexidine gluconate 20% solution	3 g
	Cetomacrogol emulsifying wax	15 g
	Liquid paraffin	6 g
	Water	to 60 g
(f)	Ichthammol	6 g
	Cetostearyl alcohol	3.6 g
	Wool fat	12 g
	Zinc cream	to 120 g

7.6

(a)	Wool alcohols	1.8 g
	Soft paraffin	3 g
	Hard paraffin	7.2 g
	Liquid paraffin	18 g

(b) Wool alcohols   4.5 g
      Soft paraffin   7.5 g
      Hard paraffin   18 g
      Liquid paraffin   45 g

7.7

(a) Menthol   3 g
      Eucalyptus oil   15 mL
      Light magnesium carbonate   10.5 g
      Water   to 150 mL

(b) Cetrimide   0.24 g
      Cetostearyl alcohol   6 g
      Liquid paraffin   60 g
      Water   to 120 g

(c) Cetrimide   0.09 g
      Cetostearyl alcohol   2.25 g
      Liquid paraffin   22.5 g
      Water   to 45 g

7.8

(a) Cetrimide   4.5 g
      Cetostearyl alcohol   40.5 g
      White soft paraffin   75 g
      Liquid paraffin   30 g

(b) Hydrocortisone   2.5 g
      Clioquinol   7.5 g
      Wool fat   25 g
      White soft paraffin   215 g

(c) Cetomacrogol emulsifying wax   12 g
      Benzyl alcohol   0.6 g
      Methyl paraben   0.92 g
      Water   26.48 g

(d) Cetrimide   0.9 g
      Cetostearyl alcohol   8.1 g
      White soft paraffin   15 g
      Liquid paraffin   6 g

(e) Oxytetracycline   1.8 g
     Zinc oxide   12 g
     Salicylic acid   3 g
     Starch   43.2 g

(f) Cetrimide   1.2 g
     Cetostearyl alcohol   10.8 g
     White soft paraffin   20 g
     Liquid paraffin   8 g

(g) Cetomacrogol emulsifying wax   45 g
     Benzyl alcohol   2.25 g
     Methyl paraben   3.45 g
     Water   99.3 g

7.9

(a) Hydrogen peroxide 20 vol   3.0 mL
     Water   12.0 mL

(b) Hydrogen peroxide 100 vol   12.5 mL
     Water   37.5 mL

7.10

     Menthol   1.2 g
     Eucalyptus oil   6 mL
     Light magnesium carbonate   3.6 g
     Water   to 60 mL
     In practice a slight excess of light
     magnesium carbonate would be used   4 g

7.11

(a) Aspirin   2.8 g
     Tragacanth   0.16 g
     (or compound tragacanth powder)   1.6 g
     Chloroform water   to 80 mL

(b) Aspirin   2.4 g
     Raspberry syrup   15 mL
     Amaranth solution   0.6 mL
     Tragacanth   0.12 g

	(or compound tragacanth powder)	1.2 g
	Chloroform water	to 60 mL

(c)

Chalk	5.4 g
Syrup	36 mL
Cinnamon water	45 mL
Tragacanth	0.36 g
(or compound tragacanth powder)	3.6 g
Chloroform water	to 180 mL

(d)

Aromatic chalk	4.5 g
Opium tincture	2 mL
Catechu tincture	2 mL
Tragacanth	0.1 g
(or compound tragacanth powder)	1.0 g
Chloroform water	to 50 mL

(e)

Sulfadimidine	11.25 g
Raspberry syrup	3 mL
Benzoic acid solution	0.15 mL
Amaranth solution	0.08 mL
Tragacanth	0.15 g
(or compound tragacanth powder)	1.5 g
Chloroform water	to 75 mL

7.12

(a)

Arachis oil	40 mL
Acacia	10 g
Chloroform water	to 100 mL
Primary emulsion:	
Arachis oil	40 mL
Chloroform water	20 mL
Acacia	10 g

(b)

Cod liver oil	35 mL
Acacia	8.75 g
Chloroform water	to 70 mL
Primary emulsion:	
Cod liver oil	35 mL
Chloroform water	17.5 mL
Acacia	8.75 g

(c) Terebene   50 mL
     Acacia   25 g
     Water   to 250 mL
     Primary emulsion:
     Terebene   50 mL
     Water   50 mL
     Acacia   25 g

(d) Cinnamon oil   45 mL
     Acacia   22.5 g
     Water   to 150 mL
     Primary emulsion:
     Cinnamon oil   45 mL
     Water   45 mL
     Acacia   22.5 g

(e) Halibut liver oil   30 mL
     Acacia   7.5 g
     Chloroform water   to 60 mL
     Primary emulsion:
     Halibut liver oil   30 mL
     Chloroform water   15 mL
     Acacia   7.5 g

(f) Liquid paraffin   25 mL
     Acacia   8.33 g
     Chloroform water   to 50 mL
     Primary emulsion:
     Liquid paraffin   25 mL
     Chloroform water   16.67 mL
     Acacia   8.33 g

(g) Olive oil   36 mL
     Acacia   9 g
     Water   to 120 mL
     Primary emulsion:
     Olive oil   36 mL
     Water   18 mL
     Acacia   9 g

(h) Calciferol   1.5 mL
     Bulking oil   8.5 mL

	Acacia	2.5 g
	Chloroform water	to 50 mL
	Primary emulsion:	
	Oils (calciferol plus bulking)	10 mL
	Chloroform water	5 mL
	Acacia	2.5 g
(i)	Peppermint oil	50 mL
	Bulking oil	50 mL
	Acacia	37.5 g
	Chloroform water	to 500 mL
	Primary emulsion:	
	Peppermint oil	50 mL
	Chloroform water	50 mL
	Acacia	25 g
	Bulking oil	50 mL
	Chloroform water	25 mL
	Acacia	12.5 g

Total chloroform water 75 mL and acacia 37.5 g

7.13

(a)	Starch	10.5 g
	Zinc oxide	12 g
	Olive oil	3 g
	Wool fat	4.5 g
(b)	Magnesium trisilicate	3.75 g
	Light magnesium carbonate	5.625 g
	Sodium bicarbonate	1.875 g
	Chloroform water, double strength	37.5 mL
	Water	to 75 mL
(c)	Starch	42 g
	Zinc oxide	36 g
	Olive oil	24 g
	Wool fat	18 g
(d)	Clioquinol	2.25 g
	Cetomacrogol emulsifying wax	22.5 g
	Chlorocresol	0.075 g
	Water	to 75 g

(e) Belladonna tincture   4.8 mL
Benzoic acid solution   2.4 mL
Glycerol   12 mL
Syrup   24 mL
Water   to 120 mL

(f) White beeswax   1.2 g
Hard paraffin   1.8 g
Cetostearyl alcohol   3 g
Soft paraffin   54 g

(g) Light magnesium carbonate   1.5 g
Sodium bicarbonate   2.5 g
Aromatic cardamom tincture   1.5 mL
Chloroform water, double strength   25 mL
Water   to 50 mL

(h) Wool fat   1.5 g
Hard paraffin   0.75 g
Cetostearyl alcohol   2.25 g
Soft paraffin   25.5 g

(i) Wool alcohols   7.2 g
Soft paraffin   12 g
Hard paraffin   28.8 g
Liquid paraffin   72 g

(j) Calamine   16.8 g
Arachis oil   72 g
Emulsifying wax   14.4 g
Water   to 240 g

(k) Cetrimide   3.6 g
Cetostearyl alcohol   32.4 g
White soft paraffin   60 g
Liquid paraffin   24 g

(l) Magnesium sulphate   24 g
Light magnesium carbonate   3 g
Concentrated peppermint water   1.5 g
Chloroform water, double strength   18 mL
Water   to 60 mL

(m) Ichthammol   1.5 g
Cetostearyl alcohol   0.9 g

	Wool fat	3 g
	Zinc cream	24.6 g
(n)	Zinc oxide	45 g
	Arachis oil	52.5 g
	Wool fat	15 g
	Water	to 150 g
(o)	Hydrocortisone	1.2 g
	Clioquinol	3.6 g
	Wool fat	12 g
	White soft paraffin	103.2 g

CHAPTER 8

8.1	**(a)** 0.80%	**(c)** 0.67%	**(e)** 0.40%
	(b) 0.25%	**(d)** 0.19%	**(f)** 1.20%
8.2	**(a)** 0.8%	**(c)** 0.48%	**(e)** 0.4%
	(b) 1.2%	**(d)** 0.2%	**(f)** 0.4%
8.3	**(a)** 3 L	**(c)** 1500 mL	**(e)** 625 mL
	(b) 750 mL	**(d)** 800 mL	
8.4	**(a)** 250 mL	**(d)** 250 mL	**(g)** 500 mL
	(b) 187.5 mL	**(e)** 200 mL	
	(c) 125 mL	**(f)** 562.5 mL	
8.5	**(a)** 0.38%	**(c)** 2%	**(e)** 0.6%
	(b) 1.2%	**(d)** 0.2%	
8.6	**(a)** 0.2%	**(c)** 1.2%	**(e)** 0.4%
	(b) 1.2%	**(d)** 0.5%	
8.7	**(a)** 600 mL	**(d)** 1500 mL	**(g)** 300 mL
	(b) 1000 mL	**(e)** 3 mL	**(h)** 625 mL
	(c) 937.5 mL	**(f)** 1125 mL	**(i)** 1000 mL

8.8	**(a)** 5 mL	**(e)** 20 mL	**(i)** 15 mL
	(b) 5 mL	**(f)** 5 mL	**(j)** 15 mL
	(c) 10 mL	**(g)** 20 mL	
	(d) 15 mL	**(h)** 15 mL	

8.9	**(a)** 5 mL	**(c)** 20 mL
	(b) 5 mL	**(d)** 15 mL

8.10	**(a)** 20 mL	**(c)** 5 mL	**(e)** 15 mL
	(b) 5 mL	**(d)** 5 mL	**(f)** 10 mL

8.11	**(a)** 0.3% w/w	**(c)** 0.5% w/w	**(e)** 1.8% w/w
	(b) 0.2% w/w	**(d)** 0.25% w/w	

8.12	**(a)** 200 mg	**(c)** 300 mg	**(e)** 200 mg
	(b) 200 mg	**(d)** 150 mg	**(f)** 195 mg

8.13	**(a)** 200 mg	**(d)** 300 mg	**(g)** 150 mg
	(b) 300 mg	**(e)** 450 mg	
	(c) 300 mg	**(f)** 150 mg	

8.14 1.5 mL

8.15 3 mL

8.16 Measure 1.75 mL, but since there is some uncertainty and it is difficult to measure, make 80 mL by measuring 2 mL

8.17 2.5 mL

8.18 1.25 mL

8.19 50 mL

8.20 75 mL required, suggest making 80 mL by using 4 mL

8.21
(a) 0.52 g	**(d)** 0.77 g	**(g)** 1.55 g
(b) 0.78 g	**(e)** 4.69 g	**(h)** 2.07 g
(c) 0.78 g	**(f)** 0.78 g	**(i)** 4.71 g

8.22

(a) Drug 1.53 g, ointment 148.47 g
(b) Drug 3.03 g, ointment 146.97 g
(c) Drug 2.54 g, ointment 97.46 g
(d) Drug 5.05 g, ointment 194.95 g
(e) Drug 0.62 g, ointment 59.38 g
(f) Drug 2.74 g, ointment 87.26 g
(g) Drug 1.01 g, ointment 48.99 g
(h) Drug 0.62 g, ointment 119.38 g
(i) Drug 0.39 g, ointment 74.61 g

8.23

(a) 25 mg/5 mL: 80 mL; 100 mg/5 mL: 20 mL
(b) 25 mg/5 mL: 133.33 mL; 100 mg/5 mL: 66.67 mL

8.24

(a) 5% ointment 15 g, 8% ointment 15 g
(b) 5% ointment 40 g, 8% ointment 20 g
(c) 5% ointment 10 g, 8% ointment 50 g

8.25

(a) 25 mg/5 mL: 40 mL; 50 mg/5 mL: 10 mL
(b) 25 mg/5 mL: 60 mL; 50 mg/5 mL: 40 mL
(c) 25 mg/5 mL: 200 mL; 50 mg/5 mL: 800 mL

8.26

(a) 5% w/w: 24 g; 7.5% w/w: 6 g
(b) 5% w/w: 24 g; 7.5% w/w: 36 g
(c) 5% w/w: 72 g; 7.5% w/w: 48 g

8.27

(a) 95% alcohol: 76.92 mL; 70% alcohol: 23.08 mL
(b) 50% alcohol: 200 mL; 95% alcohol: 50 mL

(c) 75% alcohol: 45 mL; 59% alcohol: 35 mL
(d) 20% alcohol: 88 mL; 95% alcohol: 32 mL
(e) 75% alcohol: 842.11 mL; water: 1157.89 mL

| **8.28** | **(a)** 2.3 mL | **(c)** 3.0 mL | **(e)** 2.0 mL |
| | **(b)** 1.2 mL | **(d)** 3.5 mL | **(f)** 5.0 mL |

| **8.29** | **(a)** 2.4 mL | **(b)** 2.7 mL | **(c)** 3.3 mL |

| **8.30** | **(a)** 2.20 mL | **(c)** 1.24 mL | **(e)** 2.39 mL |
| | **(b)** 5.11 mL | **(d)** 7.75 mL | **(f)** 3.60 mL |

| **8.31** | **(a)** 2.0% | **(b)** 8.89% |

| **8.32** | **(a)** 1.0 g | **(b)** 1.2 g |

8.33   0.3 g

8.34   15 mL

8.35   5 mL

8.36
(a) 937.5 mL
(b) 18.75%
(c) 2.7 mL
(d) 25 mg/5 mL: 30 mL; 50 mg/5 mL: 20 mL
(e) Drug 0.78 g, ointment 149.22 g
(f) 300 mg
(g) 95% alcohol 81 mL, 45% alcohol 69 mL
(h) 1.32 g
(i) 0.17% w/w
(j) 480 mg
(k) 0.42%
(l) 10 mL
(m) 3.67 mL
(n) 450 mg
(o) 3.15 mL
(p) 1.30 g

(q) 375 mL
(r) 12.5 mg, 2 mL
(s) 25 mg/5 mL: 160 mL; 100 mg/5 mL: 40 mL
(t) 0.4%
(u) 750 mL
(v) 5 mL
(w) 1.5% w/w
(x) 0.3%
(y) 2.5 mL to 50 mL
(z) 20 mL

CHAPTER 9

Note that there are often different ways of making triturations.
The answers given represent one method of doing the
calculation. Other answers are acceptable providing the
correct dose is contained in the final mixture.

9.1

(a) Weigh 100 mg, dissolve in 10 mL water, take 0.7 mL,
make to 35 mL with water
(b) Weigh 100 mg, dissolve in 100 mL water (required for
solubility), take 20 mL, make to 50 mL with water
(c) Weigh 100 mg, dissolve in 10 mL water, take 2.5 mL,
make to 50 mL with water
(d) Weigh 100 mg, dissolve in 10 mL water, take 0.5 mL,
make to 50 mL with water
(e) Weigh 100 mg, dissolve in 100 mL water (to allow
accurate measurement of next volume), take 17.5 mL,
make to 35 mL with water
(f) Weigh 100 mg, dissolve in 10 mL water, take 3.0 mL,
make to 50 mL with water
(g) Weigh 100 mg, dissolve in 100 mL water, take 3.5 mL,
make to 35 mL with water

9.2

(a) Weigh 100 mg drug, dilute with 900 mg lactose, take
120 mg of mixture and mix with 2.280 g of lactose to give
2.4 g total

(b) Weigh 100 mg drug, dilute with 900 mg lactose, take
150 mg of mixture and mix with 3.450 g of lactose to give
3.6 g total

(c) Weigh 100 mg drug, dilute with 900 mg lactose, take
200 mg of mixture and mix with 1.000 g of lactose to give
1.2 g total

(d) Weigh 100 mg drug, dilute with 900 mg lactose, take
100 mg of mixture, dilute with 900 mg lactose, take
800 mg of second mixture and mix with 1.600 g of
lactose to give 2.4 g total

(e) Weigh 100 mg drug, dilute with 900 mg lactose, take
100 mg of mixture, dilute with 900 mg lactose, take
300 mg of second mixture and mix with 1.500 g of
lactose to give 1.8 g total

(f) Weigh 100 mg drug, dilute with 900 mg lactose, take
120 mg of mixture and mix with 3.480 g of lactose to give
3.6 g total

(g) Weigh 100 mg drug, dilute with 900 mg lactose, take
100 mg of mixture and mix with 2.300 g of lactose to give
2.4 g total

(h) Weigh 100 mg drug, dilute with 900 mg lactose, take
500 mg of mixture and mix with 2.500 g of lactose to give
3.0 g total

(i) Weigh 100 mg drug, dilute with 900 mg lactose, take
100 mg of mixture, dilute with 900 mg lactose, take
400 mg of second mixture and mix with 2.000 g of
lactose to give 2.4 g total

(j) Weigh 100 mg drug, dilute with 900 mg lactose, take
110 mg of mixture and mix with 2.530 g of lactose to give
2.64 g total

(k) Weigh 100 mg drug, dilute with 900 mg lactose, take
140 mg of mixture and mix with 4.060 g of lactose to give
4.2 g total

(l) Weigh 100 mg drug, dilute with 900 mg lactose, take 140 mg of mixture and mix with 3.220 g of lactose to give 3.36 g total

9.3 Individual dose 45 mg, total drug is 450 mg. Use 3, 150 mg tablets, dilute to 1200 mg, pack 10 powders of 120 mg

9.4 Individual dose is 1 mg, total drug is 3 mg. Use 2 tablets, dilute to 480 mg, pack 3 powders of 120 mg.

9.5 Individual dose is 200 mg, total drug is 3600 mg. Take 12 capsules. These weigh 3816 mg. Make to 3960 mg (to produce a weighable amount), pack 18 powders of 220 mg

9.6 Individual dose is 20 mg, total drug is 420 mg. Use 9 capsules, make to a total of 2700 mg (to allow for excess of drug) and pack 21 powders of 120 mg

9.7 Individual dose is 6 mg, total drug is 84 mg. Use 9 capsules, dilute to 1800 mg (to allow for excess of drug) and pack 14 powders of 120 mg

CHAPTER 10

10.1 **(a)** 0.98 g   **(c)** 2.05 g   **(e)** 2.04 g
(b) 1.02 g   **(d)** 3.99 g

10.2 1.01 g

10.3 **(a)** 7.27 g   **(g)** 36.15 g   **(m)** 19.17 g
(b) 5.50 g   **(h)** 5.81 g   **(n)** 9.81 g
(c) 21.69 g   **(i)** 10.00 g   **(o)** 4.61 g
(d) 7.85 g   **(j)** 11.45 g   **(p)** 9.09 g
(e) 11.50 g   **(k)** 12.92 g
(f) 7.68 g   **(l)** 9.68 g

10.4

(a) Drug 1 g, base 19.09 g
(b) Drug 4 g, base 28.92 g
(c) Drug 1.25 g, base 9.17 g
(d) Drug 3 g, base 9.69 g
(e) Drug 600 mg, base 5.45 g
(f) Drug 5 g, base 16.67 g
(g) Drug 1.2 g, base 7.74 g

10.5   Hamamelis dry extract 1.2 g, zinc oxide 3.6 g, base 10.43 g

10.6

(a) Hamamelis dry extract 1.2 g, zinc oxide 3.9 g, base 10.25 g
(b) Bismuth subgallate 1.2 g, resorcinol 0.39 g, zinc oxide 0.78 g, base 5.13 g
(c) Bismuth subgallate 1.2 g, resorcinol 0.39 g, zinc oxide 0.78 g, base 5.37 g
(d) Bismuth subgallate 1.8 g, resorcinol 1.2 g, zinc oxide 1.2 g, base 10.28 g
(e) Bismuth subgallate 2 g, resorcinol 1 g, zinc oxide 2.5 g, base 17.66 g

10.7   59.33 g

10.8   25.38 g

10.9

(a) Hydrocortisone 300 mg, base 7.53 g
(b) Procaine hydrochloride 1 g, base 12.04 g
(c) Tannic acid 300 mg, base 14.24 g

10.10

(a) Procaine hydrochloride 600 mg, base 27.29 g
(b) Sulfanilamide 1.8 g, base 14.21 g
(c) Castor oil 104 mg, base 51.74 g

10.11 Morphine sulphate 118 mg, base 11.64 g

10.12 Lactic acid 1.48 g, base 47.96 g

10.13 Zinc oxide 0.59 g, base 11.17 g

10.14 Phenol 67 mg, base 67.1 g

10.15 Menthol 76 mg, base 25.17 g

10.16 (a) 1.6(2)   (c) 1.68 = 1.7
       (b) 1.17 = 1.2   (d) 5.1(3)

CHAPTER 11

11.1 (a) 14 tablets   (d) 112 tablets   (g) 126 tablets
      (b) 56 tablets   (e) 21 tablets   (h) 168 tablets
      (c) 84 tablets   (f) 56 tablets

11.2
(a) 28 tablets of 500 mg
(b) 56 tablets of 50 mg
(c) 168 tablets of 50 mg
(d) 189 tablets of 25 mg
(e) 112 tablets of 100 mg
(f) 42 of both tablets
(g) 56 of 50 mg and 56 of 100 mg tablets or 168 of 50 mg
    tablets
(h) 84 of 50 mg and 168 of 100 mg tablets
(i) 42 of 5 mg and 84 of 10 mg tablets
(j) 84 of each of 1 mg, 2 mg and 5 mg tablets, or 336 of
    2 mg tablets (4 per dose)

11.3 (a) 21 days   (c) 28 days   (e) 7 days
      (b) 7 days   (d) 14 days   (f) 14 days

11.4 (a) 105 tablets   (b) 60 tablets   (c) 168 tablets

11.5	(a) 70 mL	(d) 210 mL	(g) 210 mL
	(b) 280 mL	(e) 150 mL	(h) 1120 mL
	(c) 210 mL	(f) 280 mL	

11.6	(a) 200 mL	(b) 280 mL	(c) 630 mL

11.7

(a) 168 mL, using a 2 mL dose
(b) 35 mL using a 2.5 mL dose
(c) 84 mL using a 2 mL dose

11.8

(a) A 10 mL dose requires 280 mL
(b) A 5 mL dose requires 140 mL
(c) A 15 mL dose requires 630 mL
(d) A 10 mL dose requires 210 mL
(e) A 5 mL dose requires 150 mL
(f) A 10 mL dose requires 840 mL

11.9	(a) 7 days	(c) 21 days	(e) 14 days
	(b) 28 days	(d) 14 days	(f) 21 days

11.10 2 mg 0.1 mL, 17 mg 0.85 mL, 43 mg 2.15 mL

11.11 1 mL 10 mg, 8 mL 80 mg, 20 mL 200 mg

11.12 0.08 mL injection, 62 doses

11.13 300 mL

11.14 2400 g

11.15 100 g

11.16 200 mL

11.17 No, the range would be 30–60 g

11.18 (a) 2.85 g   (c) 3.10 g   (e) 2.95 g
         (b) 4.05 g   (d) 3.45 g

11.19 (a) 11 mg   (d) 10 mg   (g) 10 mg
         (b) 13 mg   (e) 12 mg   (h) 19 mg
         (c) 12 mg   (f) 8 mg

11.20 (a) 38 mg   (c) 223 mg
         (b) 197 mg   (d) 190 mg

11.21 (a) 36.54 units   (c) 94 mg   (e) 44 mg
         (b) 41.16 units   (d) 101 mg   (f) 42 mg

11.22 (a) 130 mg   (d) 145 mg   (g) 104 mg
         (b) 40 mg   (e) 40.11 units (h) 115 mg
         (c) 41.16 units (f) 46 mg   (i) 111 mg

11.23 Dose 525 mg, 7 capsules

11.24 17.5 g which is 35 tablets. Give, 12, 12, 11 tablets.

11.25 4 tablets per dose, 56 tablets for 1 week

11.26 Dose is 380 mg, can be taken as three 100 mg and four 20 mg capsules

11.27 2$\frac{1}{2}$ tablets per dose, 70 tablets. Instruct to divide a tablet and take half with two full tablets twice daily.

11.28 (a) 2 mL   (c) 2.8 mL   (e) 4 mL
         (b) 2.1 mL   (d) 3.3 mL

11.29 (a) 0.3 mL   (b) 0.24 mL   (c) 0.35 mL

11.30 (a) 2 mL   (c) 1.5 mL   (e) 30 mL
         (b) 1.5 mL   (d) 5 mL   (f) 7.5 mL

CHAPTER 12

12.1
(a) Young 37 mg, Clark 33 mg, BSA 53 mg
(b) Young 10 mg, Clark 10 mg, BSA 18 mg
(c) Young 25 mg, Clark 25 mg, BSA 36 mg
(d) Fried 0.8 mg, Young 0.8 mg, Clark 1.4 mg, BSA 2.8 mg
(e) Fried 20 mg, Clark 52 mg, BSA 113 mg
(f) Young 80 mg, Clark 69 mg, BSA 110 mg
(g) Fried 2.4 mg, Clark 4.8 mg, BSA 9.9 mg

12.2 By age, dose is 112.5 mg weekly; by weight, dose is 150 mg weekly. Suggest an intermediate dose such as 130 mg

12.3 24 mg daily

12.4 Age suggests ideal body weight of about 20 kg, giving a dose of 45 mg. Actual weight is about 14 kg, suggesting a dose of 30 mg, both doses 12 hourly.

12.5 Both age and weight indicate a dose of 75 mg. Dose is acceptable.

12.6 By weight, dose range is 3.8–5.7 mg. By age, dose is 7 mg. A dose around 5–6 mg could be recommended to the prescriber.

12.7 2.5 mg/kg each dose. Actual weight indicates a dose of 42.5 mg, but ideal weight for age indicates a dose of 41.25 mg. A 40 mg dose can be recommended.

12.8 From age and weight, the child is in the age range 1–5 years. Dose by weight is 7.7 mg to be taken every 4–6 hours. If given every 4 hours, the daily dose would be 46 mg, which is in excess of maximum recommended. A frequency of every 5–6 hours could be used.

12.9 **(a)** 38.4 mg   **(c)** 18.75 mg
       (b) 39. 6 mg   **(d)** 11.34 units

12.10 Dose is 37.5 mg, from 1.5 mL suspension. A total of 21 mL will be required and an oral syringe provided.

12.11 Dose is 750 mg from three 250 mg tablets. Total required 63 tablets

12.12 160 mg

12.13 Initial dose 135 mg, from 1.7 mL to be taken morning and night for 3 days. Then dose 162 mg from 2.0 mL to be taken morning and night for 3 days. Finally dose 189 mg from 2.4 mL to be taken morning and night for 14 days. Total volume 90 mL. Supply oral syringe. Doses cannot easily be obtained from capsules.

12.14 Estimated weight 29 kg. Dose 116 mg from 11.6 mL of suspension for 14 days, followed by 116 mg twice daily from 11.6 mL twice daily for 14 days. Total required 490 mL. Oral syringe required.

12.15 Assume normal weight and height (best to check), which gives body surface area 1.25 m². Dose is 750 mg twice daily (1.5 g under 2 g limit). Can be provided by three 250 mg capsules twice daily (total 84 capsules), or one 250 mg capsule and one 500 mg tablet twice daily (28 of each), or 3.75 mL suspension twice daily (total 105 mL and suitable syringe provided).

12.16 Estimated surface area 0.4 m². Dose is half 96 mg. Since tablets are 25 mg, suggest 100 mg daily dose given as two 25 mg tablets twice daily—84 tablets in total.

CHAPTER 13

13.1   (a) 500 mg   (c) 125 mg   (e) 375 mg
          (b) 500 mg   (d) 625 mg

13.2   (a) 3 g   (b) 600 mg   (c) 1 g

13.3   (a) 125 mL   (c) 125 mL
          (b) 300 mL   (d) 250 mL

13.4   (a) 225 mL   (b) 100 mL   (c) 900 mL

13.5   (a) 500 mg   (b) 125 mg   (c) 250 mg

13.6   (a) 1.25 g/10 mL   (c) 400 mg/10 mL
          (b) 800 mg/10 mL

13.7   (a) 88 mL   (d) 148 mL   (g) 104 mL
          (b) 107 mL   (e) 127 mL
          (c) 122 mL   (f) 82 mL

13.8   (a) 100 mL   (c) 20 mL   (e) 75 mL
          (b) 120 mL   (d) 105 mL

13.9   (a) 117 mL   (c) 163 mL   (e) 67 mL
          (b) 112 mL   (d) 114 mL

13.10 (a) 4.6 mL   (b) 19 mL   (c) 39.2 mL

13.11

(a) 5 mg add 19.94 mL, 30 mg add 19.64 mL, 100 mg add 18.80 mL
(b) 300 mg add 9.76 mL, 600 mg add 9.52 mL
(c) 1 g add 99.5 mL, 5 g add 97.5 mL
(d) 2.25 g add 28.43 mL, 4.5 g add 26.85 mL

13.12 0.96 mL

13.13 (a) 3.65 mL   (b) 4.95 mL   (c) 0.86 mL

CHAPTER 14

14.1   (a) 219 mg   (b) 821 mg   (c) 1276 mg

14.2   (a) 42 mg   (d) 170 mg   (g) 81 mg
           (b) 152 mg   (e) 10 mg   (h) 133 mg
           (c) 3.5 mg   (f) 27 mg   (i) 87 mg

14.3   1.299 g

14.4   1.225 g

14.5   82 mg

14.6   390 mg

14.7   (a) 3.733 g   (d) 4.394 g   (g) 3.566 g
           (b) 1.673 g   (e) 4.513 g
           (c) 4.261 g   (f) 4.474 g

14.8   (a) 4.4 mL   (b) 1.95 mL

14.9   (a) 200 mL   (d) 16 mL   (g) 10.2 mL
           (b) 80 mL   (e) 31.9 mL
           (c) 105 mL   (f) 10.7 mL

14.10 (a) 3.30 mL   (d) 1.43 mL   (g) 1.11 mL
           (b) 1.98 mL   (e) 1.80 mL   (h) 5.11 mL
           (c) 5.50 mL   (f) 3.23 mL

14.11

(a) 0.13 mL/min, 769 min (12 h 49 min)
(b) 0.5 mL/min, 1000 min (16 h 40 min)
(c) 1.6 mL/min, 313 min (5 h 13 min)

14.12

(a) 0.44 mL/min, 250 min (4 h 10 min)
(b) 5.5 mL/min, 10 min
(c) 0.67 mL/min, 94 min (1 h 34 min)

14.13

(a) 135 mL, 8 h 20 min
(b) 75 mL, 11 h 7 min
(c) 75 mL, 8 h 20 min
(d) 169 mL, 6 h 40 min

14.14

(a) 2 mL/min for 30 min, then 1 mL/min for 2 h, then
    0.5 mL/min. Latter could continue for 640 min (10 h
    40 min)
(b) 0.76 mL/min for 1 h then 0.10 mL/min for 24 h
(c) 5.2 mL/min for 30 min, then 2.6 mL/min for 2 h.
    Remainder (40 min) at 1.3 mL/min

14.15   0.84 mL/min.

14.16

(a) 20 mL in first 30 min, 160 mL after 4 h, 480 mL after 12 h
(b) 75 mL after 90 min, 125 mL after 150 min, 250 mL after
    300 min
(c) 65 mL after 60 min, 162.5 mL after 2.5 h, 260 mL after
    4 h
(d) 60 mL after 80 min, 127.5 mL after 170 min, 187.5 mL
    after 250 min

14.17   (a) 2.08 mL/min   (b) 1.39 mL/min

14.18   1.39 mL/min, finish approx. 3 p.m.

14.19   10 h, finish approx. 8 a.m. the following day

14.20   62.5 mL, finish approx. 12.30 (midnight)

14.21   Approx 5.40 p.m.

14.22   **(a)** 1.83 mL/min   **(c)** 1.22 mL/min
            (b) 1.70 mL/min   **(d)** 3.40 mL/min

14.23

(a) Add 250 mL, rate 4.17 mL/min

(b) Add 180 mL, to give 200 mL, rate 3.33 mL/min

14.24   **(a)** 17 drops/min   **(d)** 64 drops/min
            (b) 17 drops/min   **(e)** 26 drops/min
            (c) 58 drops/min

14.25   Add 250 mL, rate 56 drops/min

14.26   **(a)** 34 drops/min   **(c)** 33 drops/min
            (b) 68 drops/min

14.27   13 drops/min

14.28   First 5 min, 1.25 mL/min, 75 drops/min, then
2.03 mL/min, 122 drops/min for 5 min, then 2.80 mL/min,
168 drops/min for 5 min

CHAPTER 15

15.1   BMI = 21

15.2   BMI = 26

15.3   BMI = 30 (this patient is obese.)

15.4   1.8

15.5   Once-a-day tablet, £0.96/day

15.6   100 mg tablets, $27.00

15.7   £45.00

15.8   £11.61

15.9   IV therapy, £13.92 per day, average; oral therapy, £0.10 per day, average

15.10   £17.30

15.11   Cefazolin, £13.89; cefoxitin, £19.68; cefotan, £18.82

15.12	**(a)** 41.3%	**(b)** 43.3%	**(c)** 46.4%

15.13	£1.09	**15.21**	£5.12
15.14	£524.16	**15.22**	£4.87
15.15	£1.05	**15.23**	2.40%
15.16	£26.00	**15.24**	£3.42
15.17	£3.01	**15.25**	€2.44
15.18	£2.27	**15.26**	£8.96
15.19	£0.90	**15.27**	£5.26
15.20	41.67%		

CHAPTER 16

16.1   Mean = 128.6, median = 128, mode = 127

16.2   Mean = 304.6 mg, range = 21 mg, average deviation = 5.6 mg, standard deviation = 6.76 mg

16.3   Mean = 2.51%, median = 2.51%, mode = 2.52%

16.4

(a) 495.5 mg or 496 mg
(b) Tablets weighing ± 37 mg of the average weight fall within the designated limit. Others do not

16.5   Mean = 100 mg, average deviation = 1.65 mg, standard deviation = 2.12 mg

16.6   E

CHAPTER 17

17.1	22.7 L	**17.6**	Answer is option (b)
17.2	0.198 h^{-1}	**17.7**	Answer is option (c)
17.3	3.13%	**17.8**	Answer is option (b)
17.4	35 L	**17.9**	Answer is option (b)
17.5	35.7 µg/dL		

CHAPTER 18

18.1	C	**18.11**	A
18.2	C	**18.12**	A
18.3	D	**18.13**	B
18.4	B	**18.14**	C
18.5	D	**18.15**	D
18.6	E	**18.16**	B
18.7	D	**18.17**	D
18.8	D	**18.18**	B
18.9	C	**18.19**	D
18.10	A	**18.20**	C

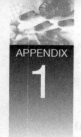
Basic arithmetic processes

DEFINITIONS

Integer	A whole number, which has neither decimal place nor fractions.
Fraction	A numerical quantity which is not an integer.
Vulgar fraction	A ratio made up of two numbers, such as $\frac{1}{2}$. This is made up of two numbers, the numerator and denominator.
Numerator	This is the number at the top of the fraction.
Denominator	This is the number at the bottom of the fraction.
Proper fraction	A fraction in which the numerator is smaller than the denominator (e.g. $\frac{3}{4}$).
Improper fraction	A fraction where the numerator is larger than the denominator (e.g. $\frac{4}{3}$).
Mixed number	A combination of integer and proper fraction. A mixed number can be produced from an improper fraction (e.g. $\frac{4}{3}$ is the improper fraction, $1\frac{1}{3}$ is the mixed number).
Decimal fraction	A number which includes a decimal point such that the numbers proceed in tenths. Often just called a decimal.
Decimal place	The number of figures to the right of the decimal point (e.g. 5.48 has 2 decimal places, 2.5397 has 4 decimal places).
Multiplicand	A number being multiplied.
Multiplier	A number by which the multiplicand is being multiplied.

| Dividend | A number which is to be divided. |
| Divisor | A number by which the dividend is being divided. |

MULTIPLICATION BY MULTIPLES OF 10

When multiplying by 10, 100, 1000 or other multiples, the answer can be obtained by moving the decimal point in the multiplicand to the right by the same number of positions as there are zeros in the multiplier. Additional zeros are added to the original number if needed.

Example A1.1
Multiply 0.24 by: (i) 10, (ii) 1000, (iii) 10 000

(i) $0.24 \times 10 = 2.4$ (there is 1 zero in the multiplier, so move the decimal point 1 position to the right).

(ii) $0.24 \times 1000 = 240.0 = 240$ (there are 3 zeros in the multiplier, so move the decimal point 3 positions to the right).

(iii) $0.24 \times 10\,000 = 2400.0 = 2400$ (there are 4 zeros in the multiplier, so move the decimal point 4 positions to the right).

Note: zeros are added as necessary to make up places where necessary. When the answer is a whole number, the decimal point may be omitted.

When multiplying by decimal fractions of 0.1, 0.01, etc, the decimal point is moved to the left by one position for each decimal place before the first number in the multiplier.

Example A1.2
Multiply 0.52 by: (i) 0.1, (ii) 0.01, (iii) 0.0001

(i) $0.52 \times 0.1 = 0.052$ (there is 1 number after the decimal point in the multiplier, so move the decimal point 1 place to the left).

(ii) $0.52 \times 0.01 = 0.0052$ (there are 2 numbers after the decimal point in the multiplier, so move the decimal point 2 places to the left).

(iii) $0.52 \times 0.0001 = 0.000052$ (there are 4 numbers after the decimal point in the multiplier, so move the decimal point 4 places to the left).

DIVISION BY MULTIPLES OF 10

When dividing by multiples of 10, the decimal point in the dividend is moved to the left by the number of zeros in the divisor. Additional zeros are added before and after the decimal point if required.

Example A1.3
Divide 56.9 by: (i) 10, (ii) 100, (iii) 10 000

(i)   56.9/10 = 5.69 (there is 1 zero in the divisor, so move the decimal point 1 position to the left).
(ii) 56.9/100 = 0.569 (here are 2 zeros in the divisor, so move the decimal point 2 positions to the left).
(iii) 56.9/10 000 = 0.00569 (there are 4 zeros in the divisor, so move the decimal point 4 positions to the left).

When dividing by decimal fractions such as 0.1, 0.001, the decimal point in the dividend is moved to the right by the number of numbers after the decimal point in the divisor.

Example A1.4
Divide 128.6 by: (i) 0.1, (ii) 0.001, (iii) 0.0001

(i)   128.6/0.1 = 1286 (there is 1 number after the decimal point in the divisor, so the decimal point in the dividend is moved 1 place to the right).
(ii) 128.6/0.001 = 128 600 (there are 3 numbers after the decimal point in the divisor, so the decimal point in the dividend is moved 3 places to the right).
(iii) 128.6/0.0001 = 1286 000 (there are 4 numbers after the decimal point in the divisor, so the decimal point in the dividend is moved 4 places to the right).

MULTIPLICATION OF DECIMALS

When multiplying decimal numbers, the number of decimal places changes. The number of decimal places produced in a multiplication is found by adding the number of decimal places in the numbers being multiplied. Thus, if two whole numbers are multiplied, there are no decimal places and none is produced in the answer. If one of the numbers has one decimal place and the other does not, the answer will have one decimal place. However, if both numbers have two decimal places, the answer will have four decimal places.

Example A1.5
Multiply the following: (i) 72×3, (ii) 7.2×3, (iii) 0.72×0.3

For each answer, the number of decimal places (dp) is shown:

(i) $72 \times 3 = 216$
    0 dp + 0 dp = 0 dp
(ii) $7.2 \times 3 = 21.6$
    1 dp + 0 dp = 1 dp
(iii) $0.72 \times 0.3 = 0.216$
    2 dp + 1 dp = 3 dp

Example A1.6
Multiply (i) 0.63×2, (ii) 0.63×200, (iii) 6.3×20

The same principle applies, but where there are zeros before the decimal point, these show as negative numbers in the calculation of the number of decimal places:

(i) $0.63 \times 2 = 1.26$
    2 dp + 0 dp = 2 dp
(ii) $0.63 \times 200 = 126$
    2 dp + $-$ 2 dp = 0 dp
(iii) $6.3 \times 20 = 126$
    1 dp + $-$ 1 dp = 0 dp

FACTORS

A factor is a number which can be divided into another number and the answer is a whole number, that is it leaves no remainder. Prime numbers are the only numbers which do not have factors. The number 14 has two factors, that is 2 and 7. Other numbers will have many more factors, for example the number 20 has factors of 2, 4, 5, 10. Two numbers may have one or more common factor. These are factors which occur in both numbers.

Example A1.7

What are the factors in the numbers 45 and 36? Are there any common factors?

Factors for 45 are 3, 5, 9, 15.
Factors for 36 are 2, 3, 4, 6, 9, 12, 18.
It can be seen that the numbers 3 and 9 are common to both lists and so they are common factors.

WORKING WITH FRACTIONS

It is a common part of solving equations that fractions are produced and require to be simplified. Particularly when working without a calculator, it is important to be able to do this efficiently. The techniques involve looking for common factors or multiplying or dividing by decimal fractions. Collectively they are commonly called simplifying or 'cancelling down' the fraction.

Example A1.8

Simplify the fraction $^{28}/_{32}$

Firstly, look for the factors of the two numbers:

Factors for 28 are 2, 4, 7, 14.
Factors for 32 are 2, 4, 8, 16.

We can see that there are two common factors, namely 2 and 4. If we divide both the top and bottom of the equation by either of the common factors, the equation will be simplified:

Dividing $^{28}/_{32}$ by 2 give $^{14}/_{16}$.
Dividing $^{28}/_{32}$ by 4 gives $^{7}/_{8}$.

These two can be converted into a decimal fraction by dividing the numerator by the denominator (see later in this appendix), giving an answer of 0.875 in both cases. The important point to note is that it is far easier to divide by 8 than by 16 or 32 without a calculator. Thus simplifying a fraction in this way enables the answer to be arrived at quickly and easily.

Sometimes, the numbers will have zeros at the end. In effect this indicates that 10, or a multiple of 10, is a likely common factor. The way of simplifying these fractions is to divide both numerator and denominator by an appropriate multiple of 10.

Example A1.9

Simplify the following fractions: (i) $^{70}/_{120}$, (ii) $^{400}/_{700}$, (iii) $^{2750}/_{4000}$

(i) In this fraction there is one zero in both the numerator and denominator, therefore each number can be divided by 10:

$$\frac{70}{120} = \frac{7}{12}$$

(ii) In this fraction there are two zeros in both numerator and denominator, therefore each number can be divided by 100:

$$\frac{400}{700} = \frac{4}{7}$$

(iii) In this fraction, there is one zero in the numerator and three zeros in the denominator. Therefore it is only possible to divide both by 10, that is 100 or 1000 are not common factors to the numerator and denominator:

$$\frac{2750}{4000} = \frac{275}{400}$$

Note: it is still possible to simplify this fraction further because there are other common factors, the largest of which is 25, which enables the fraction to be simplified to $^{11}/_{16}$.

Example A1.10

Simplify the following fractions: (i) $^{0.6}/_{0.8}$, (ii) $^{0.09}/_{0.02}$, (iii) $^{100}/_{3.5}$

When simplifying where there are decimal points, the decimals can be eliminated by multiplying by 10, 100 or other multiples as necessary to generate whole numbers in the numerator and denominator.

(i) In this fraction there is one decimal place in both the numerator and denominator, therefore multiplying each by 10 will produce integers:

$$\frac{0.6}{0.8} = \frac{6}{8}$$

This can be further simplified using the common factor 2, to give $^{3}/_{4}$.

(ii) Both the numerator and denominator have two decimal places, therefore multiplying each by 100 will produce integers:

$$\frac{0.09}{0.02} = \frac{9}{2}$$

(iii) The numerator does not have any decimal places, but the denominator has 1 decimal place. We need to multiply by a factor which will convert the largest number of decimal places into an integer, which in this case is 10. Therefore:

$$\frac{100}{3.5} = \frac{1000}{35} = \frac{200}{7}$$

CONVERTING VULGAR FRACTIONS TO DECIMALS

This process is achieved by dividing the numerator by the denominator. Some vulgar fractions will have an exact decimal equivalent, but others will not and a rounded answer will have to be given. Carrying out simplification prior to converting into a decimal will normally simplify the process. Remember when dividing, add as many zeros as required.

Example A1.11
Convert the following vulgar fractions into decimals: (i) $3/4$, (ii) $13/20$, (iii) $31/60$

(i) This is straightforward division:

$$4 \overline{)3.00} \\ \quad 0.75$$

Therefore there is a finite answer which is 0.75.

(ii) Again the division can be set up straight away because there are no factors to simplify the fraction (13 is a prime number):

$$20 \overline{)13.00} \\ \quad\; 0.65$$

This is straightforward if one is familiar with the 20-times table. However, it is possible to carry out this division in two stages, because 10 and 2 are factors of 20:

$$10 \overline{)13.00} \\ 2 \overline{)1.30} \\ \;\; 0.65$$

(iii) The denominator is a large number, so a two stage division is going to be easiest, using the factors 10 and 6:

$$10 \overline{)31.00} \\ 6 \overline{)3.1000} \\ \;\; 0.5166\ldots$$

There is no finite end to the number and therefore it has to be rounded to a number of significant figures. How many figures will be required will normally be indicated in the question or implied by the accuracy of the numbers being used. In this particular example the starting numbers are only given to 2 significant figures and so an answer to 2 significant figures is appropriate. Therefore the number would be rounded to 0.52. If, however, the starting numbers had been given as 31.0 or 60.0, this is indicating an accuracy of 3 significant figures and so the answer would have been rounded to 0.517.

Example A1.12

Convert the following fractions to decimals: (i) $^{95}/_{6}$, (ii) $22^{1}/_{2}$, (iii) $35^{5}/_{9}$ giving the answer to 2 decimal figures

(i) This is an improper fraction, but can be converted to a decimal by division as used in Example A1.11.

$$6 \overline{)95.00}$$
$$\overline{15.833\ldots}$$

There is no finite answer, so the number will have to be rounded in accordance with the question or context. This question specifies 2 decimal places, so the answer is 15.83.

(ii) This is straightforward since it is well recognized that $^{1}/_{2}$ is 0.5. With the integer given as 22, the answer will be 22.5.

(iii) $35^{5}/_{9} = 35 + \dfrac{5}{9} = 35 + 0.555\ldots = 35.555\ldots$

This number must be rounded to 2 decimal places, therefore the answer is 35.56.

SELF-STUDY QUESTIONS

Attempt these questions without using a calculator.

Multiply each number by (a) 10, (b) 100, (c) 1000, (d) 10 000, (e) 0.1, (f) 0.001, (g) 0.01:

| **A1.1** | 0.86 | **A1.3** | 0.057 | **A1.5** | 852 |
| **A1.2** | 7.3 | **A1.4** | 0.0055 | | |

Divide each number by (a) 10, (b) 100, (c) 1000, (d) 10 000, (e) 0.1, (f) 0.001, (g) 0.01:

| **A1.6** | 84.9 | **A1.8** | 5.7 | **A1.10** | 1.953 |
| **A1.7** | 703 | **A1.9** | 0.62 | | |

Carry out the following multiplications:

A1.11	91×7	**A1.19**	0.46×0.11
A1.12	5×5	**A1.20**	9.1×0.07
A1.13	46×11	**A1.21**	0.5×0.005
A1.14	91×0.7	**A1.22**	0.046×0.011
A1.15	0.5×0.5	**A1.23**	91×0.07
A1.16	4.6×1.1	**A1.24**	5×0.05
A1.17	0.91×0.07	**A1.25**	0.046×11
A1.18	0.05×0.05		

Identify the factors for the following numbers:

A1.26	20	**A1.30**	85
A1.27	72	**A1.31**	150
A1.28	192	**A1.32**	100
A1.29	135		

Simplify the following fractions:

A1.33	20/85	**A1.44**	0.75/2.5
A1.34	85/135	**A1.45**	1500/1250
A1.35	135/20	**A1.46**	1400/2500
A1.36	20/72	**A1.47**	50/120
A1.37	72/150	**A1.48**	60/150
A1.38	150/192	**A1.49**	300/200
A1.39	192/85	**A1.50**	0.6/0.3
A1.40	85/100	**A1.51**	0.09/0.3
A1.41	500/3000	**A1.52**	1.5/200
A1.42	1000/1500	**A1.53**	200/2.5
A1.43	0.05/0.02	**A1.54**	0.3/9

Express the following fractions as decimal fractions (to a maximum of 2 decimal places):

A1.55	$^4/_5$	**A1.62**	$^{31}/_{90}$
A1.56	$^7/_4$	**A1.63**	$^{11}/_4$
A1.57	$^{43}/_{25}$	**A1.64**	$^{80}/_{53}$
A1.58	$^4/_{11}$	**A1.65**	$^{90}/_{31}$
A1.59	$^6/_7$	**A1.66**	$^5/_4$
A1.60	$^1/_6$	**A1.67**	$^{25}/_8$
A1.61	$^{53}/_{80}$	**A1.68**	$^{50}/_9$

SELF-STUDY ANSWERS

A1.1(a)	8.6	**A1.7(e)**	7030	**A1.29**	3,5,9,15,
A1.1(b)	86	**A1.7(f)**	703 000		27,45
A1.1(c)	860	**A1.7(g)**	70 300	**A1.30**	5,17
A1.1(d)	8600	**A1.8(a)**	0.57	**A1.31**	2,3,5,6,10,
A1.1(e)	0.086	**A1.8(b)**	0.057		15,25,30,
A1.1(f)	0.00086	**A1.8(c)**	0.0057		50,75
A1.1(g)	0.0086	**A1.8(d)**	0.00057	**A1.32**	2,4,5,10,20,
A1.2(a)	73	**A1.8(e)**	57		25,50
A1.2(b)	730	**A1.8(f)**	5700	**A1.33**	4/17
A1.2(c)	7300	**A1.8(g)**	570	**A1.34**	17/27
A1.2(d)	73 000	**A1.9(a)**	0.062	**A1.35**	27/4
A1.2(e)	0.73	**A1.9(b)**	0.0062	**A1.36**	5/18
A1.2(f)	0.0073	**A1.9(c)**	0.00062	**A1.37**	12/25
A1.2(g)	0.073	**A1.9(d)**	0.000062	**A1.38**	25/32
A1.3(a)	0.57	**A1.9(e)**	6.2	**A1.39**	Cannot be
A1.3(b)	5.7	**A1.9(f)**	620		simplified
A1.3(c)	57	**A1.9(g)**	62	**A1.40**	17/20
A1.3(d)	570	**A1.10(a)**	0.1953	**A1.41**	1/6
A1.3(e)	0.0057	**A1.10(b)**	0.01953	**A1.42**	2/3
A1.3(f)	0.000057	**A1.10(c)**	0.001953	**A1.43**	5/2
A1.3(g)	0.00057	**A1.10(d)**	0.0001953	**A1.44**	3/10
A1.4(a)	0.055	**A1.10(e)**	19.53	**A1.45**	6/5
A1.4(b)	0.55	**A1.10(f)**	1953	**A1.46**	14/25
A1.4(c)	5.5	**A1.10(g)**	195.3	**A1.47**	5/12
A1.4(d)	55	**A1.11**	637	**A1.48**	2/5
A1.4(e)	0.00055	**A1.12**	25	**A1.49**	3/2
A1.4(f)	0.0000055	**A1.13**	506	**A1.50**	2/1
A1.4(g)	0.000055	**A1.14**	63.7	**A1.51**	3/10
A1.5(a)	8520	**A1.15**	0.25	**A1.52**	3/400
A1.5(b)	85 200	**A1.16**	5.06	**A1.53**	80/1
A1.5(c)	852 000	**A1.17**	0.0637	**A1.54**	1/30
A1.5(d)	8520 000	**A1.18**	0.0025	**A1.55**	0.80
A1.5(e)	85.2	**A1.19**	0.0506	**A1.56**	1.75
A1.5(f)	0.852	**A1.20**	0.637	**A1.57**	1.72
A1.5(g)	8.52	**A1.21**	0.0025	**A1.58**	0.36
A1.6(a)	8.49	**A1.22**	0.000506	**A1.59**	0.86
A1.6(b)	0.849	**A1.23**	6.37	**A1.60**	0.17
A1.6(c)	0.0849	**A1.24**	0.25	**A1.61**	0.66
A1.6(d)	0.00849	**A1.25**	0.506	**A1.62**	0.34
A1.6(e)	849	**A1.26**	2,4,5,10	**A1.63**	2.75
A1.6(f)	84 900	**A1.27**	2,3,4,6,8,9,	**A1.64**	1.51
A1.6(g)	8490		12,18,24,36	**A1.65**	2.90
A1.7(a)	70.3	**A1.28**	2,3,4,6,8,	**A1.66**	1.25
A1.7(b)	7.03		12,16,24,	**A1.67**	3.13
A1.7(c)	0.703		32,48,64,96	**A1.68**	5.56
A1.7(d)	0.0703				

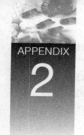

APPENDIX

2

Systems of weights and measures

INTRODUCTION

In 1960 the Système International d'Unités (SI system), based on the metric system, was adopted as the standard. Since 1969 all prescriptions in the UK have been dispensed in this system. The older imperial and apothecary systems are still found in older books and formularies. This appendix outlines the three systems for weight and volume.

UNITS OF WEIGHT

Metric (SI) system

The basic unit is the kilogram (kg), which is the mass of the International Prototype Kilogram.

Name of unit	Abbreviation	Relationship
Kilogram	kg	
Gram	g	1/1000 (0.001) kg
Milligram	mg	1/1000 (0.001) g
Microgram	µg (or mcg)	1/1000 (0.001) mg
Nanogram	ng	1/1000 (0.001) µg
Picogram	pg	1/1000 (0.001) ng

To avoid confusion between mg, mcg and ng it is advisable not to use these abbreviations in dispensing.

Imperial system

The pound (avoirdupois) (lb) is the basic unit.

Name of unit	Abbreviation	Relationship
Pound	lb	
Ounce	oz	1/16 lb
Grain	gr	1/7000 1b
		1/437.5 oz

Apothecary (troy) system

The grain is the basic standard and is the same as the
Imperial grain (gr).

Name of unit	Abbreviation	Relationship
Grain	gr	
Scruple	Ә	20 gr
Drachm	ℨ	60 gr
Ounce (apoth)	℥	480 gr
		8 drachms

Note: the imperial and apothecary ounce are not the same
weight.

VOLUME

Metric (SI) system

The basic unit is the litre (L) which is defined as 1 cubic
decimetre.

Unit	Abbreviation	Relationship
Litre	L	
Millilitre	mL	1/1000 (0.001) L
Microlitre	μL	1/1000 (0.001) mL

Imperial system

The basic unit is the pint (pt).

Name of unit	Abbreviation	Relationship
Pint	pt	
Fluid ounce	fl oz	1/20 pt

Apothecary (troy) system

The minim (ℳ) is the basic unit.

Name of unit	Abbreviation	Relationship
Minim	ℳ	
Fluid drachm	ʒ	60 ℳ
Fluid ounce	℥	8 ʒ
		480 ℳ

AMOUNT OF SUBSTANCE

The basic unit is the mole which is the amount of substance containing as many formula units as there are in 12 g of carbon-12. The formula units may be atoms, molecules, ions, etc.

Name of unit	Abbreviation	Relationship
Mole	mol	
Millimole	mmol	1/1000 (0.001) mol
Micromole	μmol	1/1000 (0.001) mmol

CONCENTRATION

Concentration can be expressed as g per L or mol per L (and multiples of these units). In dispensing, the former type of unit is normally used for drug concentration. Electrolyte concentration may be expressed as amount of substance (mol per L). In medical records and literature, mol per L is normally used.

LENGTH

The metre (m) is the basic unit.

Name of unit	Abbreviation	Relationship
Metre	m	
Centimetre	cm	1/100 (0.01) m
Millimetre	mm	1/1000 (0.001) m
Micrometre	μm	1/1000 (0.001) mm
Nanometre	nm	1/1000 (0.001) μm

General note

When expressing quantity, it is important to avoid the risk of error or misinterpretation. To reduce this it is best to avoid decimal fractions where possible. Thus, it is better to use 50 mg rather than 0.05 g. Where a decimal point is used, it should be preceded by a 0, thus it should be 0.1 g rather than .1 g.

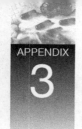

Selected atomic weights of elements

Atomic weights of elements are quoted to **4 significant figures**.

Element	Symbol	Atomic weight
Aluminium	Al	26.98
Barium	Ba	137.3
Bismuth	Bi	209.0
Bromine	Br	79.90
Calcium	Ca	40.08
Carbon	C	12.01
Chlorine	Cl	35.45
Copper	Cu	63.55
Fluorine	F	19.00
Gold	Au	197.0
Hydrogen	H	1.008
Iodine	I	126.9
Iron	Fe	55.85
Lithium	Li	6.941
Magnesium	Mg	24.31
Manganese	Mn	54.94
Nitrogen	N	14.01
Oxygen	O	16.00
Phosphorus	P	30.97
Platinum	Pt	195.1
Potassium	K	39.10
Sodium	Na	22.99
Sulphur	S	32.07
Zinc	Zn	65.39

REFERENCES

Cockcroft DW, Gault MH 1976 Prediction of creatinine clearance from serum creatinine. *Nephron* **16:** 31

Jelliffe RW 1971 Estimation of creatinine clearance when urine cannot be collected. *Lancet* **1**: 975

Jelliffe RW 1973 Creatinine clearance bedside estimate. *Annals of Internal Medicine* **79**: 604

FURTHER READING

Ansel HC, Stoklosa MJ 2001 *Pharmaceutical Calculations, 11th Edn.* Lippincott Williams and Wilkins, Baltimore

Aulton ME 2002 *Pharmaceutics: The Science of Dosage Form Design, 2nd Edn.* Churchill Livingstone, Edinburgh

British National Formulary, current edition. British Medical Association and Royal Pharmaceutical Society of Great Britain, London

British Pharmacopoeia Commission. *British Pharmacopoeia, current edition*. The Stationery Office, London

Gunn C, Carter SJ 1965 *Cooper and Gunn's Dispensing for Pharmaceutical Students, 11th Edn.* Pitman Medical Publishing, London

Hall GD, Reiss BS 2001 *Appleton and Lange's Review of Pharmacy, 7th Edn.* McGraw-Hill

Mousa AAM, Abahussain EA 2003 *Medical Statistics, 4th Edn.* Kuwait University Press, Kuwait

National Heart, Lung and Blood Institute 1998 *Clinical Guidelines on the Identification, Evaluation and Treatment of Overweight and Obesity in Adults*. National Institutes of Health Publication No. 98-4083 Available at: http://www.nhlbi.nih.gov/guidelines/obesity/bmio_tbl.htm accessed 8 November 2004

Rees JA, Smith A, Smith B 2000 *Introduction to Pharmaceutical Calculations*. The Pharmaceutical Press, London

Reynolds JEF. *Martindale: The Extra Pharmacopoeia, current edition*. The Pharmaceutical Press, London

Royal Pharmaceutical Society of Great Britain 1979 *The Pharmaceutical Codex, 11th Edn.* The Pharmaceutical Press, London

Royal Pharmaceutical Society of Great Britain 1994 *The Pharmaceutical Codex, 12th Edn.* The Pharmaceutical Press, London

Royal Pharmaceutical Society of Great Britain 2004 *Medicines, Ethics and Practice – A Guide for Pharmacists, 28th Edn.* The Pharmaceutical Press, London

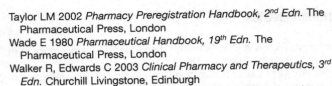

Taylor LM 2002 *Pharmacy Preregistration Handbook, 2nd Edn.* The Pharmaceutical Press, London

Wade E 1980 *Pharmaceutical Handbook, 19th Edn.* The Pharmaceutical Press, London

Walker R, Edwards C 2003 *Clinical Pharmacy and Therapeutics, 3rd Edn.* Churchill Livingstone, Edinburgh

Winfield AJ, Richards RME 2004 *Pharmaceutical Practice, 3rd Edn.* Churchill Livingstone, Edinburgh

Index

absorption, drug, 239
acacia powder, 80
accuracy, 4–5
acquisition costs, drug, 213–16
'ad', quantity value preceded by, 68
additives and additional materials (in medicines)
  intravenous, 185–9
  master formulae with, 79–82
adsorbents, 80
age
  of child and dose, 161–2, 162–4
  creatinine clearance and, 245
alligation method, 103–7
allowable discount, 213
amounts see quantities
answers
  approximating, 7
  estimating, 6–7
  reasonable, 8
antibiotics, reconstitution, 171
apothecary (troy) system
  volume, 309
  weight, 12, 308
approximation, 7
area under the plasma concentration—time curve, 243
arithmetic
  basic processes, 3–4, 4–6, 298–304
  definitions of terms, 297–8
atomic weights, 14
  various elements, 311

average(s)
  calculated see mean
  positional see median; mode
average deviation, 226–7, 228
average wholesale price, 217–19
avoirdupois system see imperial system

balances, 119
bases, suppository/pessary, 127
  displacement see displacement value
  water-miscible, 130–1
BMDP (BioMedical Data Processing Package), 235
body height/weight/surface area see height; surface area; weight
body mass index calculation, 205–8
branded and generic drugs, cost differential between, 210–11
bulk density, 53

°C (Celsius), 20
calculators
  necessary use, 4
  problems created by, 3
capsules, dose required, 141
Celsius scale, 20
Centigrade (Celsius) scale, 20
charges see payments
chi-squared test, 231–2
child doses, 161–70
Clark's rule, 163

clearance rate, creatinine, 149, 244–6
Cockcroft–Gault equation, 245, 246
colligative properties of solvent, solute altering, 181
compartmental modelling, 239–40
computers, statistical analysis, 234–5
concentrated waters, 30, 101–2
concentration(s), 25–39, 95–118, 309
  changing the, 95–118
  of drug in fluid compartments, 239
    area under the plasma concentration–time curve, 243
    fall to half its value, 240–1, 241
  molar, in calculation of isotonicity, 183
  volumes, measure of, 19
confidence intervals, 229, 230
contingency table, 231
conversion tables, weights and volumes, 13, 19
co-payment, 218
correlation, 233
corticosteroids, topical, dose, 146–7
cost (of drugs), 208–19
cost–benefit analysis, 208–9
cost differential
  between branded and generic drugs, 210–11
  between different drugs, 210
  between dosage forms and routes of administration, 211–12
  between dosing regimen, 212
  between treatment options, 212–13
cost–effectiveness analysis, 209
cost–minimization analysis, 209–10

creams, dose, 146
creatinine clearance rate, 149, 244–6
cutaneous preparations, dose, 146–7

data, statistical, 223–4
  software packages for analysis, 235
decimal fractions (decimals; decimal numbers)
  of 0.1/0.01 etc.
    division by, 299
    multiplication by, 298
  definition, 297
  multiplication of, 299–300
  vulgar fractions converted to, 303–4
decimal place, definition, 297
degrees (temperature), 20
degrees of freedom, 227
  Student's t distribution, 230
denominator, definition, 297
density, 53–7
  drug, and its displacement value, 128
  of liquids, 53–7
  of solids, 53
density factor, water-miscible bases, 130, 131
dermatological preparations, dose, 146–7
deviation, 226–8
  average, 226–7, 228
  standard see standard deviation
dilution, 79, 95, 96–102
  equation, 96–102
    complex dilutions, 107–9
discounts, 213–16
displacement values (in suppositories), 79, 128–9, 131
  definition, 128
  determination, 132
  more than one drug, 130
  published values, 128–9

displacement volume when reconstituting powders, 173–5, 185
distribution (of drug), 239
  in one compartment model, 240
  volume of, 242
distribution(s) (frequency), 224
  central tendency in, measures, 224–5
  normal see normal distribution
  t (Student's), 230–1
  variation in see variation
dividend, definition, 288
division
  in conversion of vulgar fractions to decimals, 303–4
  by decimal fractions of 0.1/0.01 etc, 299
  by multiples of ten, 299
divisor, definition, 288
dosage forms, 141–6
  amount required, 141–6
  cost differential between, and routes of administration, 211–12
  liquid see liquid
  solid, 141–4
dosage regimen, 141
  cost differential between, 212
dose(s), 139–70
  daily divided dose, 140, 141
  daily dose, 140
  definition, 139–40
  intravenous injections, 152–3
  paediatric, 161–70
  required for prescription, 141–6
  scheduling of administration see dosage regimen
  single dose, 140
  suitability of, 147–52
  total dose, 140
  weekly dose, 140
dose range, 140
drip chamber, 189–90

drop volume (in drip chamber), 189–90
drugs
  different forms, 41–51
  displacement of base by see displacement value
  dose see dosage; dose
  oral, powders for reconstitution, 171–9
  parenteral see parenteral solutions
  pharmacoeconomics, 208–19
  pharmacokinetics, 239–47
  see also medicines

economic aspects of drugs, 208–19
elderly, creatinine clearance, 245
electronic balances, 119
elements
  atomic weights see atomic weights
  symbols, 311
elimination, drug, 239
  by kidney, 244
  rate constant, 240
emulsions, 59, 80
equivalents, 16, 30–4
  solutions, 30–4
errors/mistakes
  reducing risk of, 8–9
  rounding, 6
esters, 43–4
estimating an answer, 6–7
external preparations, dose, 146–7
eye drops, isotonic, 182

°F (Fahrenheit), 20
factors, 300–1
Fahrenheit scale, 20
fees see payments
females, creatinine clearance, 244
fiftieth percentile, 225
first order kinetics, 240–3
flavoured waters, 30, 101–2
fluid compartments, 239–40

fluid ounce, avoirdupois (imperial) vs apothecary (troy), 12, 309
forms of drugs, 41–51
formulae, master, 67–93
fractions, 301–3
  decimal see decimal fraction
  definitions of various types, 297
  improper, 297
  proper, 297
  simplifying, 301–3
  vulgar see vulgar fractions
freezing point depression, 182–3, 184
frequency distributions see distributions
Fried's rule, 162–3

gelatin and glycerol base, 130
generic and branded drugs, cost differential between, 210–11
giving sets, 189
glycogelatin, 130
grains, 12, 308
gram, 11, 307
gram equivalent, 16

half-life, 240–1, 241
height
  in body mass index calculation, 205–8
  in body surface area calculation, 150, 165
  in paediatric dose calculation, 162
  see also length
hydrates, 41, 44–5
hydrogen peroxide, amount in solutions, 19
hypertonic solutions, 182
hypotonic solutions, 182

imperial (avoirdupois) system
  conversion tables (to/from other systems), 13, 19
  length, 19
  volume, 12, 308–9
  weight, 12, 307–8
improper fraction, definition, 297
infant doses, 162–3
infusion see parenteral solutions
ingredients in medicine
  amounts see quantities
  changing the concentration, 95–118
  master formulae, 67–93
  percent mark-up on cost of, with prescriptions, 216–17
injections, parenteral solutions for see parenteral solutions
integer, definition, 297
international units, 18
intravenous medicines and injection see parenteral solutions
ion(s), gram equivalent, 16
ionic weight, 14
isotonic solutions, 181–5

Jelliffe equation, 245, 246

kidney, drug elimination, 244
kilograms, 307
  body weight in
    body mass index calculation, 205
    dose based on, 149–50
kinetics of drug handling, 239–47

legal issues, different forms of drugs, 41–2, 45–7
length, units/systems of, 19–20, 310
  conversion tables, 19
  see also height
linear regression, 233
liquids
  density, 53–7
  dilution see dilution
  dose required, 144–5
    fractional doses for oral liquids, 146

liquids (*cont'd*)
  in master formulae, 75
  measuring equipment, 119
  see also solutions
list price, 213–14
litre, 12, 308
lotions, dose, 146

macrogols, 131
males, creatinine clearance, 244
mark-up, percent (prescriptions),
      216–17
*Martindale: The Extra
      Pharmacopoeia*, 67
master formulae, 67–93
mean, 224–5
  deviation from (=average
      deviation), 226–7, 228
median, 225
medicines
  additional materials, 79–82
  changing the concentration,
      95–118
  ingredients in *see* ingredients
  parenteral *see* parenteral
      solutions
  trituration from manufactured
      medicines, 123–4
  see also dosage; dose; drugs
men, creatinine clearance, 244
metre, 310
metric and SI systems
  conversion tables (to/from
      other systems), 13, 19
  differences between the two
      systems, 11
  length, 19, 310
  volume, 12, 308
  weight, 11–12, 307
micropipettes, 119
milliequivalent (mEq), 16, 30
minim, 309
mistakes *see* errors
mixed number, definition, 297
mode, 225
molar concentrations in calculation
      of isotonicity, 183

molar solutions, 30–4
mole, 14, 30, 309
  subdivisions and multiples, 15,
      309
molecular units, 14–18, 309
molecular weight, 14
mould calibration, suppositories,
      127–8
multiplicand, definition, 297
multiplication
  by decimal fractions of
      0.1/0.01 etc, 298
  of decimal numbers, 299–300
  by multiples of ten, 298
multiplier, definition, 297

net cost, 213–14
nomogram for surface area
      calculation, 165–6, 167
non-proprietary (generic) and
      branded drugs, cost
      differential between, 210–11
normal distribution, 228
  important values in, 230
  standard, 228, 230
  unit, 228, 230
numbers
  accuracy of expression, 4–5
  decimal *see* decimal numbers
  mixed, definition, 297
  rounding *see* rounding
  sense of, 6
  significant figures, 4
  see also fractions
numerator, definition, 297
nutrition, total parenteral, 193–5

obese children, dose, 164
oil-in-water emulsions, 80
ointments, dose, 146
one compartment model, 240
opioid drugs, 46
oral drugs
  cost differential between
      parenteral and, 211–12
  powders for reconstitution,
      171–9

oral syringe, 146
order of magnitude, 12
osmolarity, serum, in calculation
    of isotonicity, 183
osmotic pressure, 181–2
ounce, avoirdupois (imperial) vs
    apothecary (troy), 12, 308
    see also fluid ounce

paediatric doses, 161–70
parenteral solutions
    (predominantly
    intravenous), 181–203
    cost differential between oral
        therapy and, 211–12
    doses, 152–3
    infusion of, 185–95
        additives, 185–9
        rate of, 189–93
        for total parenteral nutrition,
            193–5
    one compartment model
        assuming IV injection,
        240
    powders for reconstitution,
        171–9, 185
    tonicity, 181–5
parts, 29–30, 72–4
    alligation method, 103–7
    in displacement values, 128
payments (fees and charges)
    private prescriptions, 216–19
    professional services, 217,
        218
Pearson correlation, 233
percentages, 25–9, 75–9
    of adult dose for children of
        different ages, 162, 163
    in dilution equations, 96–7
    percent mark-up
        (prescriptions), 216–17
    suppositories prescribed by,
        131–2
    weight in volume see weight in
        volume

percentile, 50th, 225
pharmacoeconomics, 208–19
pharmacokinetics, 239–47
pint, 12, 308, 309
pipettes, 119
plasma, area under the
    concentration–time
    curve, 243
pocket calculators see
    calculators
pound (avoirdupois), 12, 307,
    308
    body weight in, dose based
        on, 148
powders
    reconstitution in solutions,
        171–9, 185
    trituration for, 120–3
prescriptions
    dose required for, 141–6
    pricing, 216–19
    see also medicines
price, list, 213–14
pricing, prescription, 216–19
private prescriptions, payment
    for, 216–19
probability values, 230
professional fee, 217, 218
proper fraction, definition, 297
proportion, simple, scaling of
    quantities by, 69
proprietary (branded) and
    generic drugs, cost
    differential between,
    210–11
pump driver, 189

quantities/amounts, 11–24
    of ingredients in
        medicine/preparation
        list of (=master formulae),
            67–93
        for total parenteral nutrition,
            194
    molecular units, 14–18, 309

quantities/amounts (*cont'd*)
    systems of weights of
        measures, 11–12, 19–20,
        307–10
    see also dose

range, 226
ratios, 25–6
    emulsions, 81
raw data, 223
reasonable answer, 8
recipe (master formulae), 67–93
reconstitution (powders in
        solution), 171–9, 185
Registration Examination
    mock paper, 249–55
    RPSGB attitude to calculations
        in, 1, 2
regression, 233, 234
relative molecular mass, 14
relative standard deviation, 227–8
renal elimination, 244
rounding, 5–6
    errors, 6
routes of administration, cost
        differential between
        dosage forms and,
        211–12
Royal Pharmaceutical Society of
        Great Britain (RPSGB)
        Registration Exam *see*
        Registration Examination

salts, 42–3
sampling variation, 229
SAS (Statistical Analysis
        System), 235
saturation solubility, 59, 60
scaling factor, 70
scatter diagrams, 233, 234
semi-solids, dilution, 95
sense of number, 6
serum osmolarity in calculation
        of isotonicity, 183

SI system *see* metric and SI
        system
significant figures, 4
simple proportion, scaling of
        quantities by, 69
single discount equivalent,
        214–15
skin preparations, dose, 146–7
sodium chloride solutions for
        attaining isotonicity, 182
software, statistical, 235
solids
    density, 53
    dilution, 95
    dose required of solid dosage
        forms, 141–4
    in master formulae, 75
solubility, 59–66
    factors influencing, 60
solute altering colligative
        properties of solvent, 181
solutions
    of concentrated (flavoured)
        waters, 30, 101–2
    concentration *see*
        concentration
    molar and equivalent, 30–4
    parenteral *see* parenteral
        solutions
    powder reconstitution in,
        171–9, 185
    tonicity, 181–5
    trituration for, 119–20
    see also liquids
solvent, solute altering colligative
        properties of, 181
SPSS (Statistical Package for the
        Social Sciences), 235
standard deviation, 227–8, 229
    in normal distributions, 228, 229
    relative, 227–8
standard errors, 229
standard normal deviate, 230
standard normal distribution,
        228, 230

STATA (statistical analysis package), 235
statistical analysis, 223–37
  computer software packages, 234–5
steroids, topical, dose, 146–7
strengths
  mixing two materials of different, 96
  of solid dosage forms, 141
Student *t* distribution, 230–1
suppositories and pessaries
  bases *see* bases
  mould calibration, 127–8
  prescribed by percentages, 131–2
surface area (patient)
  calculation, 150, 165, 167
  dose based on, 150–1
    paediatric, 162, 163, 165–6
suspension, suspending agents, 79–80
syringes
  intravenous injection, 152
  oral, 146

t distribution, 230–1
tablets, dose required, 141
tabulation of data, 223–4
temperature, 20
ten, multiples of
  division by, 299
  multiplication by, 298
'to', quantity value preceded by, 68
tonicity of solutions, 181–5
topical preparations, dose, 146
total parenteral nutrition, 193–5
trade-name (branded) and generic drugs, cost differential between, 210–11
trituration, 79, 95, 119–25
  from manufactured medicines, 123–4

for powders, 120–3
for solutions, 119–20
troy system *see* apothecary system

unit(s), 18
  doses involving, 151–2
unit normal distribution, 228, 230

variation, 225–8
  measures of, 225–8
  sampling, 229
volume(s) (measure of concentration), 19
volume(s) (measure of space occupied)
  in dilution equations, 96–102
  displacement, when reconstituting powders, 173–5, 185
  drop (from drip chamber), 189–90
  in master formulae, 69–72
  units/systems of, 12, 308–9
    conversion between various systems, 13
  see also weight in volume
volume in volume
  in master formulae, 75
  percentage (%v/v), 27–8
volume of distribution, 242
vulgar fractions
  conversion to decimals, 303–4
  definition, 297

water
  presence or absence in molecule, 41
  for reconstitution
    sterility, 171, 173
    volume, 173–4
water-in-oil emulsions, 80
water-miscible bases, 130–1
waters, concentrated, 30, 101–2
weighing, 119

weight(s)
  body
    adult dose based on,
      148–50
    paediatric dose based on,
      162
    in surface area calculation,
      150, 165
  in body mass index
      calculation, 205–8
  in master formulae, 69–72
  units/systems of, 11–12, 307–8
    conversion between various
      systems, 13–14

weight in volume
  in master formulae, 75
  percentage (%w/v), 19, 27
    in dilution equations, 96–7
weight in weight
  in master formulae, 75
  percentage (%w/w), 26–7
women, creatinine clearance,
      244

Young's rule, 163

Printed in the United States
By Bookmasters

Printed in the United States
By Bookmasters